PSORIASIS

The Rowland Remedy

I dedicate this book to all the families of my clients who by their support have made so many successful treatments possible.

PSORIASIS

The Rowland Remedy

John Rowland

JAVELIN BOOKS
POOLE · DORSET

First published in the UK 1986 by Javelin Books,
Link House, West Street, Poole, Dorset, BH15 1LL

Distributed in the United States by
Sterling Publishing Co., Inc.,
2 Park Avenue, New York, NY 10016

British Library Cataloguing in Publication Data

Rowland, John
Psoriasis: the Rowland remedy.
1. Psoriasis
I. Title
616.5'2606 RL321

ISBN 0 7137 1676 2

Typeset by Lovell Baines Print Ltd., Newbury, Berkshire, England.

Printed and bound in Great Britain by the Guernsey Press Co. Guernsey, C.I.

Contents

Acknowledgements

I would like to thank my colleagues, family and friends for their help in compiling this book, in particular Angus Thomas, BSc, CChem, FRSC.

Foreword

Through the years working at the Naturopathic Private Clinic as a chiropodist, I have come into contact with many of John Rowland's patients who suffer from psoriasis and, to this day, I never cease to be amazed at the dramatic results John achieves. Over a relatively short period of time, people who have suffered with psoriasis for years are able to enjoy life, including sports and pastimes which they have long been unable to pursue.

John Rowland trained as a horticulturist and, during this training, became interested in the herbal properties of plants, so much so that he subsequently qualified from the Faculty of Herbal Medicine as a herbalist and graduated to the General Council of Consultant Herbalists.

John has worked closely with such leading herbalists as John Napier and Dr William Mellor and, with this background and his acquired knowledge of herbalism, he is without doubt Europe's finest herbalist.

People travel from all over the world to attend his clinics and they are all treated alike with complete impartiality, which always puts them at ease. His achievements with patients young and old are a result of his dedication to herbalism. Through this book, John Rowland offers new hope to all psoriasis sufferers, and I consider it an honour and privilege to write this foreword.

Stephen Anwyl MSSCh

Preface

Recently, when travelling from Blackpool to my London clinic, I entered into conversation with a young medical student who took great pleasure in telling me that herbalists were no longer referred to as alternative practitioners but as 'complementary' practitioners working in complementary medicine. This is progress indeed, a far cry from the dismissive attitude of many older members of the medical profession, and I hope that the progress demanded by the public at large towards greater flexibility within the medical profession will continue at a rapid pace.

The student showed great interest in my work and found many of the topics that we discussed of interest, particularly my approach to psoriasis. He had just been studying dermatology and had found that there had been very little change in the standard treatment for psoriasis for a great many years. Today's orthodox treatments are still as reliant as ever on anti-mitotic substances (which slow the rate of division of diseased cells) and steroids, as anybody with the condition will know.

He also showed the same surprise at the amount of discipline and organisation that exists in our field of medicine, as did some postgraduate student doctors who recently visited my clinic from a local hospital.

People who visit herbalists tend to have chronic conditions which have failed to respond to conventional medicine as prescribed by their doctor, and it is often in desperation that they turn to someone like me. They are sometimes so disillusioned that they have very little confidence left in their ability to cope with life and the first thing I have to do is restore their confidence, both in themselves and in what they can expect from herbal treatment.

It usually surprises people, but certainly reassures them, to know that the training of herbalists today is rigorously controlled. In the UK, it is undertaken by the Faculty of Herbal Medicine and by the National Institute of Medical Herbalists, each body providing academic training leading to diploma qualifications. At the end of the course, there is a period of practical instruction from experienced medical herbalists. Both organisations are flourishing and ensure by their efforts that the high esteem in which British herbalism is held throughout the world is continued.

It should be pointed out that it is still not a legal requirement in the UK to be qualified before one may practise herbal medicine, although moves are being made in this direction. Because of this, I strongly advise any client seeking help to ask whether or not the practitioner they have in mind is qualified. The letters to look out for are MRH or MNIMH. The first signifies that the holder is a registered medical herbalist who has undergone training with the Faculty of Herbal Medicine: this is the training section of the General Council and Register of Consultant Herbalists (address on p.125). The letters MNIMH signify that the practitioner has undergone training with the National Institute of Medical Herbalists and has become a member of that body (address on p.125). Both organisations have graduates working in Canada, Australia and New Zealand.

In the UK, the growth of herbal medicine was given a boost by the introduction of the Medicine Act (1968). The previous Act had been lax enough to allow the release onto the market of drugs such as thalidomide, and so the new Act was passed. It gave the opportunity for the British Herbal Medicine Association, whose members include such well-known practitioners as Hugh Mitchell, Fletcher

Hyde, David and Tony Hampson and Marjorie and Kenneth Robinson, to have a clause included that ensured that medical herbalists had the freedom they required to develop their profession.

Since the new Medicine Act, the same stringent controls that are placed on the pharmaceutical industry are placed also on herbal preparations. The rigid quality control demanded by the Department of Health and Social Security (DHSS) or the Ministry of Agriculture, Fisheries and Food (MAFF) in the UK and the Food and Drug Administration (FDA) in the USA has undoubtedly improved the standard of preparations on the market, though the controls are not without their drawbacks for herbalists: the main problem is that most herbal knowledge is accumulated by observation rather than by clinical trials and, in order to satisfy the regulations covering the marketing of herbal preparations, one has to show scientifically how they work on the body's metabolism.

This is also more difficult to evaluate when following an holistic self-care system such as the one that I am describing for psoriasis, so I would welcome letters from you telling of your experiences whilst on the programme. The address of my clinic is on p.125.

The fact that herbal medicine is based on knowledge accumulated over thousands of years is something I touch on when reassuring prospective clients about the respectability of the profession. Even today, much information is passed on from one individual to another and I, for example, have the privilege of having known some of the herbalists of an earlier generation who were responsible for keeping herbalism alive in Britain during a difficult period. C. Abbott, F. Power, J. Napier, E. Hackett and my good friend and colleague Lawrence Brimelow are some of them.

In an initial interview with my client, I have also to point out the limitations of herbalism. If I were involved in a car crash and required surgery of some kind then I would go to a surgeon for treatment; if I had any condition that would best be treated by the use of antibiotics then I would, and do, consult my local general practitioner. If, however, a condition is one of toxaemia or, like that of psoriasis, arthritis, hypertension, colitis or asthma, one of degeneration, then it is almost always worthwhile trying an holistic approach – herbal medicine integrated into a total health programme similar to the one explained in this book.

It may also be useful to continue some drugs prescribed by a doctor, as in an holistic approach it is not the means, but the end, which counts, and that end is eventual restored good health. The Chinese attitude to medicine is such that the patient can receive either herbal or orthodox medicine or, if appropriate, both. Nobody gets upset because of professional pride; each profession is respected for the contribution it is making to the individual's total health programme.

I look forward to the day when, in the West, professional prejudice is put aside for the benefit of the individual and hope that the information given in this book is a start in the right direction.

Certainly the information can be used in a number of ways. The holistic self-care programme which is described is designed specifically for the treatment of psoriasis and can be followed at home, preferably in consultation with a family doctor. As an integral part of the treatment plan, detailed advice is given on how to eat sensibly (the Rowland Remedy Food Guide) and this can be used as a basis for healthy living generally. The final part of the book is a straightforward reference section, dealing with herbs, vitamins, minerals and trace elements and various important foodstuffs, and gives details of their sources, composition and health-giving properties. Taken as a whole, the book will give the reader an insight into the use of herbalism as part of an holistic form of treatment and also into the influence herbalism is having on modern medicine and society in general.

John Rowland
Cleveleys, 1985

Introduction to Herbalism

Medicine has throughout its history been dependent upon nature as its prime source of medicaments. Today this dependence still remains, with all the major pharmaceutical companies intently sifting through the world's folklore trying to discover a new plant-based substance which would match the many successes of the past. These successes include morphine, which to this day is the most successful painkiller that we have.

The theory and principles that I put forward in this book are not new. Plant medicine in the cultures of ancient China and Egypt was one of the major sciences and, thousands of years later, I am presenting you with the same principles which they used in an effort to create a situation in which the body can heal itself. Our advantage over the Ancients is that we have the accumulated knowledge, ancient and modern, Eastern and Western, on which to base our treatment programmes.

As recently as the beginning of this century, almost all the medicines prescribed by doctors had their origins in the plant kingdom, many being dispensed in the form of extracts, or pills, or infusions, as we suggest in this book. Herbal medicine was trusted because it had evolved over thousands of years of trial and error.

When the pharmaceutical industry discovered its ability to synthesise drugs from plant sources and mineral elements, herbal medicine lost favour because it was slower in action than the new, convenient and immediate preparations. The effect of the new drugs, even if dubious in relevance to the ailment, was to satisfy both doctor and patient, in the short term at least, as something was being achieved immediately.

The position of herbal medicine was further weakened by the discovery of antibiotics, probably the greatest gift to mankind this century, responsible for alleviating more suffering, and saving more life, than any other form of medicine. (It is of interest to note, however, that, if the massive need for penicillin had not arisen during World War 2, it had already been planned to extract and market the antibiotic properties of garlic on a commercial scale.) You need only stand in the outpatients' department of any hospital for a few minutes to be convinced of the need for the drugs and surgery of allopathic medicine, as orthodox Western medicine is termed, and yet there is a movement throughout the world rejecting many of these drugs in favour of a revival of interest in plant medicine. There is a desire for mild, natural cures which can be used in conjunction with an holistic approach to self-care.

I think this about-turn on the part of the public all over the world is the result of two basic factors. The first is that people are in general better educated than formerly and feel confident of their ability to take responsibility for their own health as far as is possible; the second is that the side effects of many drugs used in allopathic medicine are, or can be, much worse than the original condition for which they have been prescribed. These drugs have evolved in part because of a natural desire on the part of the public for a miracle pill in times of illness, with the medical profession believing, and allowing the public to believe, that such a thing is possible. The pharmaceutical industry seems to have been able to convince everybody, mainly by glossy advertising, that miracles can indeed be worked.

The public, however, has slowly come to realise that the only miracle that exists is the human body, and that it is the body's own defences that we should be helping wherever possible. The search for mild, effective medicine which has minimal side effects, is non-habit forming and which can be used in a self-care system is the dominant cause of a world-wide resurgence of interest in herbs, vitamins, minerals and alternative therapies, a movement now so great that throughout the world it is being referred to as the 'green wave'.

Herbal medicines are natural substances derived from plants, whereas many allopathic drugs are synthetic chemicals. This is not the case with all of them, however, and many well-known orthodox medicines which have stood the test of time are derived from the plant kingdom. Countless people throughout the world owe their lives to an ornamental flower called foxglove (*Digitalis purpurea*), which doctors prescribe to correct irregular heart beats, strengthen the heart muscle contractions and prevent congestive heart failure. It acts by maintaining a healthy balance between the sodium and potassium in the heart cells.

A major success story of hospitals specialising in the treatment of cancer has been the breakthrough in the management of leukaemia and Hodgkin's lymphoma by the use of alkaloids. Alkaloids are nitrogenous substances occurring naturally in plants. They possess marked physiological properties and are often medicinally valuable. Some plants contain a very large number of alkaloids, and two of the sixty alkaloids present in the Madagascar periwinkle are being extracted: leukocristine which is active against leukaemia, and vincaleukablastine which is active against Hodgkin's lymphoma. They act by interfering with the assembly of tubulin, a protein which is essential to the structure and form of the cell, and so they slow down the rate of division of the cancer cell.

The fact that plant derivatives are so successfully used in some substances in orthodox medicine raises the question of why herbal medicine should so casually be dismissed out of hand by many practitioners of this allopathic medicine! It often comes as a surprise to people that the original source of aspirin was the willow bark which contains salicylic acid, its synthetic form being acetyl salicylic acid.

On the subject of pain, it is interesting to know that the herb curare, which the South American Indians use as poison in their blowpipes, has its use in most hospitals today; it contains an agent called tubocurarine which surgeons use to relax the muscles prior to an operation.

Rauwolfia serpentina has long been used by herbalists to reduce blood pressure. The alkaloids which do the work have been isolated and are in use all over the world helping people to fight hypertension.

Two herbs in particular have had a dramatic effect on the state of the world today. The first of these in cinchona, which is the source of quinine and associated agents used in the treatment of malaria. Without this drug, explorers and pioneers would not have survived very long, and progress into uncharted wilds would have taken much longer to accomplish. Missionaries regarded cinchona as an indispensable agent in their medicine chest and it quickly became known as Jesuits' bark, a name which survives today.

The other herb that has had such a wide-reaching effect on the society we live in is the Mexican wild yam, from which we obtain an agent called diosgenin, a precursor for many of the steroid-based preparations available today, not least of which is the contraceptive pill with all its connotations of freedom for women.

Herbal medicines are natural substances derived from plants which are often used by the plant for purposes such as defence against attack by insects or being eaten by other members of the animal kingdom. They are substances manufactured by the plant for that particular purpose and are therefore outside the main biochemic pathways of proteins, fats and carbohydrates. The current orthodox approach is to isolate these secondary plant products and try and define their specific action on the body, thence creating a new drug which is a purely chemical substance. The herbalist differs radically in his approach, using the whole herb, or whole herbal extracts, in the belief that the secondary plant products are better administered to the body in the balance put there by nature. This is termed as being in its synergistic form, which herbalists believe will give the body all the benefits of the whole range of substances to be found in each plant. There are fewer side effects from this method of use but most of the benefits, particularly when used in conjunction with an holistic treatment programme such as the one advocated in this book. The variety of substances contained in a herb balances what might be the harsh effect of a powerful individual chemical. The plant *Ephedra* is used, for example, to treat asthma: the chemical ephedrine, which is the ingredient active against asthma, has the side-effect of raising the blood pressure, but other constituents of the plant, included in herbal preparations, counter the effect of the ephedrine on the blood pressure. In the use of ephedrine in orthodox medicine, high blood pressure is risked and, if encountered, treated by yet another drug.

It is reasonable to suppose that secondary plant products will make valuable contributions to medicine in the future. There can be as many as a hundred secondary substances in any one plant and, given that there are over 350,000 known species of plant in the world, and so far we have only a cursory knowledge of about 10,000 of them, there is remarkable scope for research.

The argument put forward by the pharmaceutical industry is that, by using their methods, they can reproduce the chemicals found in plants more accurately and therefore dispense more accurate doses than the herbalist, particularly as a plant's ingredients vary from season to season or even month by month.

The herbalists' reply to this is that the isolated chemical from the plant, and subsequent reproduction in the laboratory, has left out many of the other ingredients in the plant that act as a safeguard, as we have seen with *Ephedra*.

To a herbalist it does not make sense to give a specific chemical for a specific ailment as a drug cannot confine itself to any one specific action. It may well do the job for which it was prescribed but, at the same time, it will have travelled into other areas of the body, such as the brain, heart or lungs, where the reaction may not be beneficial. Such reactions are known as side effects and in many cases are worse than the original condition for which the drug was prescribed. They can include blurred vision, diarrhoea, rashes, dizziness, fainting and palpitations.

Whilst herbs are much slower in their action, they are without doubt much safer and this, we herbalists maintain, is because the active principle of the herb is aided by the other agents which are present so that they are in harmony with nature – of which, of course, you and I are a part.

To help in this field, the World Health Organisation has established an Institute in Rome. Many universities and teaching hospitals around the world are helping with research and herbalists are contributing information. This pool of knowledge must help to advance the cause of natural medicine greatly in the coming years.

Part 1
About Psoriasis

1 What is Psoriasis?

There are over 30 million known cases of psoriasis in the world today and it is fair to assume that there are millions of unreported cases. It is a skin condition of a chronic inflammatory nature and is characterised by itchy red patches which become covered with loose, silvery scales. It has the unsightly appearance that people associate with contagious diseases and, although it is not contagious, the appearance may be one of the reasons why the psychological effects of the disease are very frequently worse than the condition itself. The double-sided nature of the problem, coupled with its widespread distribution adds up to a lot of misery. This is compounded by the fact that orthodox medicine, though it will treat the symptoms, regards the condition itself as incurable.

Any part of the body surface can be affected, but the most common sites are the scalp, forearms, elbows, knees and legs. To a lesser extent, it occurs on the chest, abdomen and the soles of the feet. When it occurs under the finger- or toe-nails, the nails become discoloured and loosened and may eventually be lost.

The cause of psoriasis has remained a mystery, although it has long been regarded as a constitutional disorder. Doctors content themselves with alleviating the prime symptom, the itching, with potentially dangerous steroid drugs, which in long-term use render the skin paper-thin. For a sufferer to be told he has an incurable ailment, particularly one which is unsightly, does nothing to help the psychological problem and, for a young person, can be especially depressing.

When people come to me for treatment my first task is to restore their confidence in the fact that they can be cured and to encourage them to lead a normal life, not covering up the affected areas but exposing them to the elements which will aid the recovery process. I have persuaded many miserable young people to have the courage to go bare-armed and bare-legged into sports and leisure activities.

CAUSES

THE ROWLAND THEORY

The skin has many roles, one of the main ones being elimination, the removal from the body of toxic substances. Another major role is to carry any excess heat or energy from the cells in the interior of the body to the surface, and to conduct or radiate it to the atmosphere. To achieve this, the skin has a considerable number of blood vessels which dilate on warm days or after strenuous activity. The manifestation of this is the flushed face, or the blush if the excess energy has come from some emotional factor such as confusion or embarassment. Flushing is caused by the blood vessels enlarging to allow a greater volume of blood more exposure to the surface, enabling the blood to discharge its excesses more quickly and thus allowing the body to regain its equilibrium.

It is my theory, the one on which I have based many hundreds of successful treatments, that the cause of psoriasis is the body producing too much energy in the cells, this energy requiring constant release through the skin and putting a strain on the skin with which it cannot cope. The sites at which this takes place become those showing the symptoms of the condition we call psoriasis.

If we accept this theory, then to counteract and cure the condition we need to take four simultaneous courses of

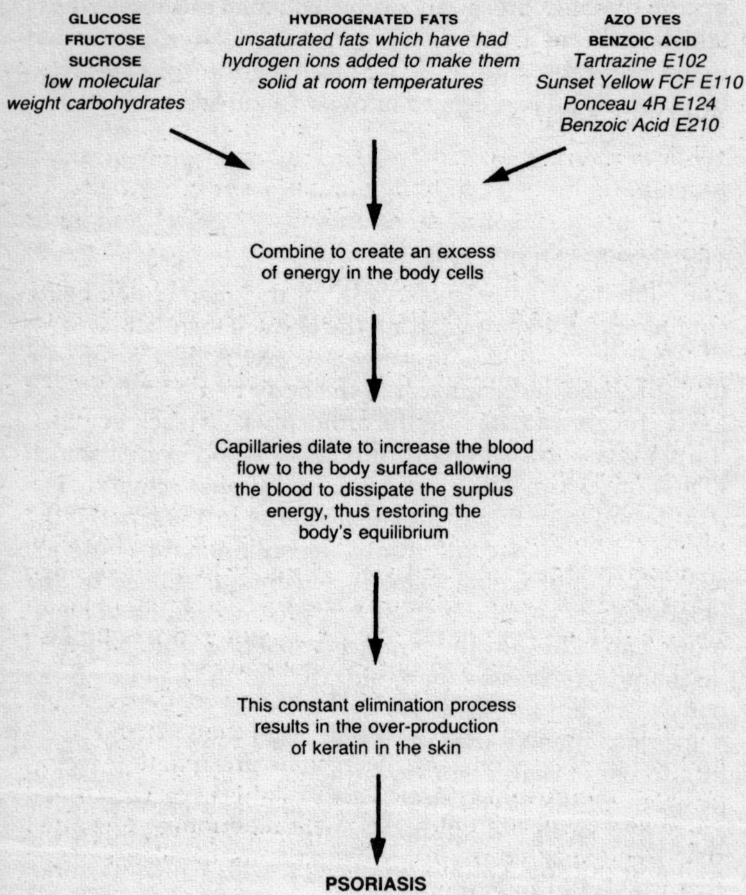

Figure 1. The Rowland Theory as to the cause of psoriasis.

action: improve the peripheral circulation; remove the causes of excess energy in the cells; detoxify the body and create a condition whereby the body can adjust and heal itself. The herbal medicinal approach to this is discussed in Chapter 3 and the methods by which we achieve these aims are discussed in detail in Part 2.

PREDISPOSITION

While certain people have a definite inbuilt predisposition to psoriasis it needs an unfavourable environmental factor to precipitate the clinical condition. The first and most important factor, in my observation, is poor diet and inherited dietary habits. It can often be seen through many generations that a particular dietary habit has been passed down – two sugars in a cup of tea or coffee for instance, or an excessive amount of fat in the recipes that are passed from one generation to another. We shall deal in much more detail with dietary habits in the treatment section but please keep this point in mind.

The second major cause in my clinical observation is that of some kind of trauma. One of the first successful treatments that I achieved was with a girl who had fallen off her horse 6 years previously and this had brought about the condition. Another person had suffered a whiplash injury and a subsequent outbreak of psoriasis.

The different stories related by my patients about traumatic situations in which they have found themselves, and which may well have been their precipitating factor, are so numerous that I could easily fill this book with them. However, I will content myself with mentioning one other that frequently crops up, with patients of all ages, and that is surgical operations.

Increased stress is the next factor that seems to precipitate the condition in a lot of people. I am of the opinion that stress plays a role in all disease and should be looked at in any holistic treatment programme. I recall a builder whose business was in such a financial mess that the mere mention of the bank manager's name was sufficient to start off that familiar itch which is often the start of a new area of psoriasis.

Sudden bereavements in the family are often the stress factor, as are examinations. It is definitely the case with this group of people that either time or the removal of the cause of stress is necessary for a successful treatment of the condition.

Hormonal imbalance has a marked effect on psoriasis, in particular at childbirth, when the condition often disappears, only to make a further reappearance within the first year after the birth.

Infection is another precipitatory cause. There is clear evidence to show that streptococcal pharyngitis has a role in the manifestation of guttate psoriasis of childhood, for example, and there are many others.

Side effects of some drugs are another common precipitatory factor, and here we have to be particularly careful in our diagnosis. Many eruptions may be mistaken for psoriasis when they are, in fact, the direct side effect of a treatment for some other condition. The use of methyldopa, gold or lithium salts, and the anti-malarials mepacrine and chloroquine can, and often do, aggravate any psoriasis that is already present.

TYPES OF PSORIASIS

Psoriasis manifests itself in eight different ways and, for interest, we will now describe each type. The holistic approach to treatment and control can be used to combat all forms of psoriasis but it should be mentioned here that, whilst all forms of the condition improve through the use of this programmed treatment, it is considerably more successful with some than others; I shall deal with these

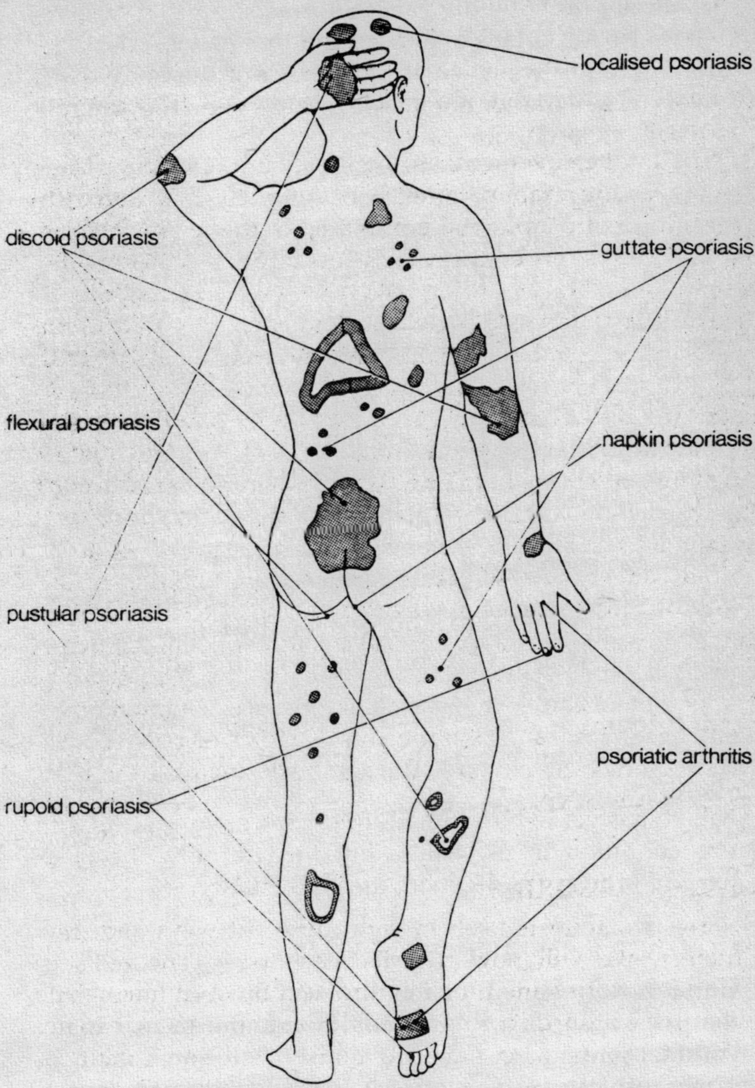

Figure 2. Common sites of psoriasis on the body.

details as I describe the various forms.

It is also important to understand that psoriasis is varied in many other ways, such as the area of the body that it covers or whether or not it always appears on the same site or changes location.

DISCOID PSORIASIS

Discoid psoriasis is by far the most common type of psoriasis in adults and is easily recognisable. It manifests itself as plaques (platelike areas) which are covered by loose silvery scales and is often so clearly defined as to be palpable. The white silvery scales may be easily detached through scraping, but this often provokes bleeding. The smaller areas often grow and join up with other areas to form distinctive patterns on the surface of the skin. The elbows, knees, lower back and edges of the scalp are the favourite sites for discoid psoriasis.

Discoid psoriasis is the type which responds most readily to the treatment programme described in this book. I cannot emphasise enough to you that this system is worthwhile following if you want to control and clear this type of psoriasis.

It is found in about 2% of the population of Europe and North America but is less common in Third World countries where a Western style of life, particularly eating habits, has yet to be adopted. I now see many Asians with this condition in my clinics but to date only one black person, who is third generation in the UK.

GUTTATE PSORIASIS

Guttate psoriasis is probably the next most common type that I see after discoid psoriasis. It is found mainly in my young clients who have previously had some form of upper respiratory infection, one in particular being streptococcal pharyngitis. This condition is, however, occasionally present in adults. The programme of treatment is highly successful but I have experienced difficulty in keeping children off sugar, which is a necessary part of the treatment.

The condition is characterised by a uniform rash of papular eruptions (small elevations of the skin which do not form pus) which are mainly found upon the trunk and limbs, as opposed to discoid psoriasis.

FLEXURAL PSORIASIS

Flexural psoriasis is found in the folds of the body, beneath the breasts and in the ano-genital area. The plaques are similar to those found in discoid psoriasis but, because of their location on the body, they are of smooth appearance, with a slightly glazed look about them which is due to the friction they encounter. This condition is often found in the elderly although it also occurs in many young people. The success of the programme depends entirely upon the general state of health of the individual.

I recall a young school teacher who, some years ago, had the condition in his ano-genital fold. This was affecting his ability to father children due to a low sperm count, which I attributed to the psoriasis generating too much heat around the scrotum, thus reducing his fertility. This would seem to have been the case because, as soon as we cleared his psoriasis, his wife became pregnant.

NAPKIN PSORIASIS

Napkin psoriasis is often found in children who have an hereditary predisposition to the condition. It is often a difficult problem with a young child but one which responds well to the programme, particularly if all the family change their eating habits. If the child is still only on milk then the milk or preparation used should be based on soya milk. If the child is solely breast-fed, the mother's diet should conform to the programme.

PUSTULAR PSORIASIS

Pustular psoriasis is often a condition of the middle-aged rather than the young, although it may be a side effect of certain types of orthodox treatments in which case it may affect any age group. It is charactised by small yellow pustules which appear in the middle of psoriatic skin, in particular on the soles of the feet or palms of the hand. In some cases just the pustules are present with no other evidence of psoriasis. Due to the rapid changes which can occur in this type of psoriasis, and the subsequent constitutional disturbance, I always advise my patients to liaise closely with their own doctor whilst following my treatment programme. A patient's doctor is in the best position to know whether or not the condition had been brought about by injudicious use of some topical treatment or drug therapy and is better able to advise on how to discontinue it. He can also diagnose whether the condition is the form of pustular psoriasis called 'rupoid'.

PSORIASIS OF THE NAILS

There is one form of psoriasis with which I have had only a limited amount of success, and that is where it affects the nails. It does seem that, whereas the treatment programme is very successful in most forms of the condition, the nails present a particular problem; to me, this seems to be the result of some complication, possibly fungal or bacterial, which helps perpetuate the condition for its own benefit.

PSORIATIC ARTHRITIS

Psoriatic arthritis is a condition in which psoriasis is combined with many of the complications of rheumatoid arthritis but in a localised area, and rarely reaching the full severity of this crippling condition.

LOCALISED PSORIASIS

Localised psoriasis is where only one or two patches, mainly of discoid psoriasis, manifest themselves. Often these patches are mistakenly diagnosed because they are limited in number. They can occur in unexpected areas, such as the tongue or on the glans penis, and are often very persistent. In my experience, where the condition has manifested itself on an unusual area of the body that person is much more inclined to follow the holistic programme vigorously and therefore more successfully than the person whose localised psoriasis is in the scalp and may well be passed off as dandruff.

2 The Orthodox Medical Approach

Very little has changed for many years in the orthodox medical approach to the control and treatment of psoriasis. It is still based on topical treatments, although recently a systemic approach has been tried using certain drugs which have contributed little to the patient and in some cases have been dangerous. The topical treatments used are based mainly on agents such as coal- or wood-tar extracts, dihydroxyanthranol or corticosteroids, on shampoos with a detergent base, and on ointments which contain oil of cade, salicylic acid and, occasionally, sulphur.

The tar extracts seem to me to be reasonably successful in controlling the irritating aspects of the disease but rather messy. They seem to work because of their anti-mitotic action, i.e. slowing down of the rate at which the cells are dividing in the area affected by the psoriasis.

Dihydroxyanthranol (Dithranol in the UK; Anathralin in the USA) is very popular because it is effective in the localised control of the condition and it is not as messy as many of the tar derivatives. It is also a stronger anti-mitotic. A major problem is that it acts as an irritant to unaffected parts of the skin and thus has to be incorporated in a dilute form when used in an ointment or paste.

For the more severe cases of psoriasis, patients often have a course of treatment either in hospital or as outpatients on a day-care basis. This can be as often as every 6 months or once a year and a regime called the Ingram regime is used as a form of treatment. This is often quite successful in clearing the condition, particularly discoid psoriasis, in about a month. Alas, it is only a brief respite, as the condition very quickly returns.

The use of corticosteroids has been popular for some time now, particularly in flexural psoriasis, as they are less messy to use than the tar or dihydroxyanthranol preparations and they are non-irritant. However, long-term use of corticosteroid preparations is not favoured due to the enormous number of side effects, the most common one in my experience being skin fragility, which not only makes the condition much worse but has an emotional effect on the sufferer as well.

On the subject of emotion, it should be noted that most orthodox treatments do show consideration for the social and psychological needs of the patient. This is a very necessary part of any treatment of psoriasis, whether it be in the form of the orthodox approach or the method of holistic self care, such as the one that we are advocating.

In the UK, the medical profession seems reluctant to use a system of treatment such as the one I suggest. Although many doctors have combated the condition in themselves by such treatment they do not seem to use it with their patients. Perhaps they have less confidence in their patients' perseverance and strength of will than I have.

I know that this is not the case in many countries and certainly I have received enquiries from members of the medical profession in the USA, Saudi Arabia, Bolivia, Malta and Spain. These enquiries are often prompted by clients who have visited my London clinic, been successful in following the programme and have so impressed their doctors at home that they have written or telephoned for an exchange of information.

Now that I am publishing my method of treatment, I am looking forward to the time when it is one of the standard approaches to the treatment of the condition in hospitals and I would certainly be interested to take part in organised projects in a controlled environment.

3 The Herbal Approach

We have seen on p.21 my theory that the main environmental factor which triggers off the inherited predisposition to psoriasis is too much energy being produced in the cells. This then begs the all-important question: 'What causes this excess of energy that overloads the natural body function?'

More often than not, one of the first observations one makes when meeting sufferers from psoriasis in a clinical situation is that their general health is good. The second is often that the client is intelligent, but inclined to be headstrong. This suggests that psoriasis could be a clinical manifestation of a healthy body's response to factors such as poor habits and stress. If this is the case, then the control of psoriasis should be a simple matter of correcting the poor eating habits which are causing the excess of energy and of paying attention to the stress factor. In my experience, the problem is caused by too high an intake of the following food substances:

1. The lower-molecular-weight carbohydrates, i.e. sugar – glucose, sucrose and fructose.
2. Hydrogenated (hard or saturated) fats.
3. Additives such as azo dyes, benzoic acid derivatives and monosodium glutamate.

Any one, or a combination, of these substances are, in my opinion, responsible for the cellular hyperactivity which eventually results in the manifestation of psoriasis. Why should this be? Let us look firstly at the problem of a high intake of sugar.

SUGAR INTAKE

In nature, one of the most sugar-rich foodstuffs that we come across is the apple, a subject that has been familiarly used to illustrate a point ever since Adam and Eve; and I, too, will take it as an example. Let us say that, more or less, the apples that are on sale throughout the world are non-toxic, natural produce, and it would seem reasonable to suppose that our digestive systems are well equipped to deal with such items.

Now, 1 teaspoonful of sugar is the equivalent of two apples. Some people, then, consume the equivalent of six apples every time they have a cup of tea. In fact, apart from these daily drinks which may represent forty or fifty apples, other foodstuffs on many people's diets contain high quantities of sugar. This could be the equivalent of another sixty or seventy apples, which would bring us to a possible 120 apples a day!! You will readily see that if you were to follow a natural diet it would be somewhat unbalanced!

It is for this reason that all or as much as is possible of sugar in the refined form of sucrose, glucose or fructose be avoided whilst on the treatment programme. The prime source of carbohydrates should be from the more complex forms such as bread, rice or cereals. (Note, however, that people with this type of skin disorder are often sensitive to corn products and this is the reason why these gain a high percentage in the Rowland Remedy Food Guide – see Chapter 7.)

Let us again go back to the apple as the example of the sort of foodstuff on which nature intended our bodies to exist and keep this in mind whilst we take a mental look at our own diet and the products that are on sale in the supermarkets. You will see that you are surrounded by an abundance of foodstuffs that are virtual power packs and which will provide the body with far more energy than it actually requires.

THE FOOD INDUSTRY AND FOOD PROCESSING

The Western food industry is one of the most highly organised and sophisticated and, in the most part, I feel that it has done an excellent job of providing an abundance of food to meet the ever-increasing demand; if some of these products are used in moderation in your diet then there is little problem. They should be enjoyed, as the body is easily able to cope with most foodstuffs in moderation. However, it is important to make good use of fresh, unadulterated foods in your diet and to reduce the amount of packaged, ready-made 'junk' food and other processed food.

What sometimes happens is that the body becomes overloaded with some of the ingredients used regularly in processed food and many people are developing a sensitivity to this cumulative effect and this is often the trigger factor in psoriasis.

Let us look for a moment at the problem of the food manufacturer. He has to make a product that sells, which means that it has to have appeal, and so he may well use a food colour in his recipe to make it more attractive. He must pay attention to the time which it takes for his product to get from his mixing pot onto your table – via the wholesaler, the retailer and your shopping bag. He may well feel that this process is going to take some time and so will put a preservative into his recipe to keep it edible until it reaches you. During the processing of any foodstuff, the fresh flavour of most of the ingredients is lost and so the food scientist may well decide to add monosodium glutamate, an agent which enhances what flavour is left after processing. Should the product contain fat, the manufacturer will often include hard fat in his recipe so that the product will not melt on the shelves. Chocolate bars are a particularly good example of this sort of use of hard fats.

There are, of course, other considerations but those

mentioned above are central to the issue of what we should eliminate from our diets in the early stages of the treatment programme – not only sugars, but also hard fats, preservatives such as benzoic acid, colours such as azo dyes and also flavour enhancers such as monosodium glutamate.

I made the point a little earlier that in moderation none of these agents would harm the body as the body's elimination processes would easily be able to cope. The problem is the cumulative effect of a regular intake of any one of these products by the individual over long periods of time. They build up and eventually make the user sensitive to even the smallest amounts. In other words the user becomes allergic to the substance and has various subsequent manifestations to that allergy – such as psoriasis.

It is important to clear your body of these toxic substances and to allow its natural healing ability to work on the ailments which they have caused. This is the holistic approach. Wherever possible, then, you should eat raw foods or foods that are fresh before cooking. These will be in accord with nature's balance and so are right for maintaining your good health as *you* are part of that natural balance.

HOW HOLISTIC TREATMENT WORKS

In a nutshell, the general concept of holistic treatment is to create a condition, by means of diet, fasting, hydrotherapy, vitamin and mineral therapy, herbal medicine and any other therapy that can make a contribution, whereby the body's own healing process can work. We are creating a programme of treatment that includes as many known agents and therapies that the body may require to heal itself. As Hippocrates recognised, all those years ago, 'the body is the prime physician'.

In this book, I am explaining the Rowland Remedy relevant to psoriasis: it is a successful way of controlling this condition providing you have the necessary life force and determination to follow the programme through. It is one of forty different programmes, called the Rowland Remedies, which are an accumulation of clinical observations and handed-down knowledge from my predecessors at the naturopathic private clinic which I run.

The concept of the programme is simple: you first detoxify the body by eliminating from your diet as many of the foods as possible that may be causing your toxic condition and, at the same time, you set about clearing away what is already there. You fast every seventh day and have special baths three times, and then twice a week in between the fast days, in addition to your normal baths. After the special baths, you apply a blend of oils to the affected areas.

To ensure that you are following the programme properly, we insist on a stipulated breakfast and lunch, but the evening meal is left very much to your own discretion. You are, however, given a guide to what you may or may not eat at this meal. This is called the Rowland Remedy Food Guide and you will find it on p.70. Having sorted out the diet and general eating habits, so that the body is not only detoxifying itself but also regenerating, we try to help it along by the use of health foods, vitamins and minerals and herbal medicine. These are listed fully in Part 3 of this book.

It should be mentioned that undertaking your self-care treatment does not mean that you are no longer your general practitioner's patient, but the fact that you are assuming more responsibility for your own good health should leave him more time to help you with counselling, and it is to be hoped that he will be interested in the progress you are making.

DETOXIFICATION

One of the first things that one must learn when beginning a self-care system of treatment is the principle of elimination and what is meant by the detoxification process which is so basic to the success of the programme. Fundamental to this is the fact that the body has four means of elimination: by faeces via the large intestine; by passing urine via the kidneys; by perspiration via the skin, and by exhalation by means of the lungs.

When the body's four means of elimination are not working properly, toxaemia arises and this becomes the basis of most degenerative diseases. Simple forms of toxaemia are coped with by evacuation (by diarrhoea or vomiting) or by biliousness when the liver returns toxins to the intestine via the bile duct. A more insidious form of toxaemia is when the liver is unable to cope with the poison and allows it to enter the bloodstream.

At this point, the body is just about coping in eliminating the excesses, but to do this it has first to have stimulated the endocrine glands to release some of their hormones in order to reinforce the elimination process. If the body has to do this on a regular basis then an endocrine imbalance is often the outcome. In effect, the constant strain put upon the body in having to eliminate toxins results in the body becoming 'run down'.

This is the basis for most degenerative disease, because when the body's defences are down the virus or mycotoxin can get a hold. Sometimes nutrients are not available to the organs of the body so that more cells die than are created and so we get an aging or degeneration of that organ.

The first conditions to make themselves known are the minor ailments, the odd ache or pain and that feeling of being one degree under and not on peak form. After a period of time these minor ailments manifest themselves into various forms of arthritis, hypertension, various skin conditions such as psoriasis and eczema and various internal inflammations, such as bronchitis and colitis.

So what causes toxaemia? It depends on the particular susceptibility of the individual, but it could be alcohol, sugar, artificial food colourings, preservatives, drugs or one of many others. Apart from these, there are over 2,000 chemicals and additives that we may come into contact with in our daily lives without our knowledge – such things as polishes, paints and glues, detergents, inks and so on. Stress can be another cause of toxaemia, often the last straw for the body's defences. One person will be more at risk from one particular toxin than another, and it is for this reason that an individual self-care system makes such good sense in the treatment of degenerative diseases.

What then is the best way to help the body use its own natural detoxifying methods? How can we best aid the processes of elimination?

The first thing to do, to ease the process of excretion, is to ensure that there is plenty of dietary fibre in our meals. Diets with a high fibre content have received a lot of publicity recently (though it should be said that nature-cure enthusiasts were until recently lone voices advocating this form of treatment) and it is easy to find out which foods are good in this respect. Wholewheat bread, whole grains and legumes, and plenty of fruit and vegetables are the prime factors. The Rowland Remedy Food Guide ensures that the intake of dietary fibre is adequate. The importance of fibre in the diet is that it acts rather like blotting paper when passing through the alimentary canal, taking up a lot of the debris and waste products. There is also the added benefit that it normalises the peristaltic action of the alimentary canal so that constipation is avoided.

After ensuring that we have sufficient dietary fibre, then we must look at the intake of fluids to ensure that the kidneys are not being over- or underworked. Remember that the kidneys are the blood's filters and the second of our four means of elimination. It is vital that we achieve the right quantity and quality of fluids in our treatment programme. I recommend lemon juice and water, or cider vinegar and water, to start the day, also the grape juice and water 24-hour fast every seventh day. Remember that water is nature's solvent and so, in the main, drinks based on water should be taken: these could be herbal teas such as chamomile, peppermint, rosehip, nettle or comfrey – there are many to experiment with, such as parsley piert or dandelion which also makes a delicious coffee. I make this point about water-based drinks because I often find patients drinking juice-only when on the programme and, though juices are permitted, they should not be taken in excess.

The next area of elimination is the skin and its function of perspiration. It takes only a moment's thought to realise that the skin is the largest organ of the body. It has many physiological functions, but the one that we are most concerned with here is the ability to perspire and in so doing reduce the body's toxic build-up. This natural ability should be encouraged to the utmost and we achieve this in the programme by the use of hydrotherapy – the special baths.

These special baths should be taken at least three times and later twice a week. The sea salt which they contain combines many natural elements and has beneficial properties, not least of which are those of healing and antisepsis. The French are great supporters of thalasso-therapy (the treatment of disease by sea bathing and sea air) and they have shown how many people who are suffering with varying diseases can be helped by effective use of the sea's natural powers. We are not all in a position to get to a warm coast at a moment's notice, but we can add sea salt to our bath water and bring some of the sea's beneficial powers to our homes.

The ingredients of the special baths are discussed fully

on p.39. The general principle is that they should stimulate free perspiration. It is advisable to take your bath late, just before bed, when, after applying the oils to the affected areas, you should wrap yourself in a bath robe to both aid and absorb the perspiration. The next day you will be pleasantly surprised at the invigorating effect of the bath and be ready to tackle your condition again.

Cider apple vinegar is added to the bath because a normal healthy skin is slightly acidic, the acidity coming in the main from the skin's secretions from the sebaceous glands which form a mantle to protect and lubricate the skin. The pH (hydrogen potential) of the skin is normally around 5.5. This shows that it is mildly acidic and, at its best, well protected by its acid mantle. The bacteria with which the skin is constantly coming into contact cannot live on an acid surface. It follows therefore that a skin which is too alkaline is going to be more prone to infection without this natural barrier. It is important, therefore, to achieve the right balance and not go too low on the pH scale. Too high an acid level will also cause the skin to be sensitive. With this information you should be able to vary the quantity of cider apple vinegar that you put into your bath a little to meet your own requirements.

The fact that 98% of known germs cannot survive in sea water for longer than 48 hours suggests that the addition of sea salt to your bath must be beneficial in clearing any unhealthy condition of the skin. Chamomile flowers, boiled, are the next addition; the benefits of these are described on p.87. Oats, the same rolled porridge oats that you eat, stop the skin becoming too taut.

The fourth method by which the body may eliminate toxins is by exhalation. We are all familiar with the smell of garlic on the breath or the person suffering with halitosis due to a gastric complication. The breath odour is caused by the body using the lungs as one way of detoxifying itself. It is with this in mind that I recommend deep breathing exercises and aerobics if you are agile enough – but only under supervision, plenty of walking, which is my favourite, and swimming if your condition allows.

You will now have a basic idea of how detoxification works and will have begun to understand the importance of aiding this process when on a total health programme. Not only do we gain the benefit of a better oxygen supply to the bloodstream, and thereby the cells, but we also rid the body of the toxic build-up which is necessary before we can begin to make progress on the healing programme.

Remember that an holistic programme is based on three premises. The first is to provide the body with all the nutrients that it could possibly need to put itself into good health. The second is to detoxify, removing all the poisons and accumulated debris from the system. The third is to improve the circulation so that the above two processes can work fully, with the cells receiving the nutrients and the waste products being carried from the cells and eliminated.

To achieve this threefold aim, we make full use of herbal medicine, vitamin and mineral supplements, hydrotherapy and exercise in an effort to create a condition in which the natural healing processes of the body can work to our best advantage.

Part 2
The
Rowland Remedy

4 The Dietary Concept

In the creation of my treatment programme, I had several basic premises which I would like you to understand. Later in the book, I deal with individual foods, vitamins, minerals and herbs, but here I would like to outline the fundamental concept at the heart of the dietary part of your programme.

A good balance of amino acids, the body's basic building blocks, is essential; from this it will be able to synthesise its proteins. Secondly, a natural emulsifier is required to prevent the build-up of fats in the arteries. Thirdly, we should create as nearly as possible what I like to call a 'ninety-two element diet': a diet comprising all the elements of which the earth, of which you and I are a part, is composed. Fourthly, every seventh day we should undertake a 24-hour fast. Finally, we should look at the problems created by sophisticated convenience foods.

Combining the above four principles with our modern knowledge about the effects of individual foodstuffs and elements on particular functions of the body, we can come up with a practical general guide as a basis for our diet programme. This guide reduces to an eight-point plan and, if you keep this in mind, you will not go far wrong in selecting suitable foods for yourself. Until you are completely familiar with the composition of the foods you eat, however, it is difficult to be sure that your diet is perfect in all respects and it is for this reason that, on the programme, the breakfast and lunch menus are stipulated, leaving only the evening meal to your own discretion. You are asked only to follow the general guidelines and the eight-point plan which is as follows: high potassium content; low sodium content; low sugar content; low saturated fat content; high fibre content; high pantothenic acid (Vitamin B_5) content; rich sources of nutrients; known peculiarities of certain foods.

Very briefly, the reasons for these criteria are as follows. Potassium is essential to the body and one of the main agents we are striving to increase in our health programme. Often the body's potassium level is depleted, mainly by the excessive use of sodium, sugar and caffeine, by using diuretics too often, or by the factor so commonly underlying countless diseases – stress. People with arthritis, hypertension, leukaemia, heart disease, epilepsy and diabetes all have a depleted potassium level, often with a correspondingly high sodium level. Most of the body's potassium is found in the cells, with a small amount in the body fluids and bloodstream. It has many roles to play, of which an important one is to help maintain a normal heart rhythm; others are the maintenance of muscle tone and the formation of extra bone, although its precise role in this is not fully understood. Further information on potassium can be found on p.113.

At one time, there was a higher proportion of potassium than sodium in our diets and, indeed, the body adapted many of its own mechanisms to retain sodium: one of the functions of the kidneys is to ensure that the minerals are in the correct balance. However, there is such a high level of sodium in our present-day diets that our bodies are being overloaded with this mineral. In the Rowland Remedy Food Guide we try to redress the balance in our food intake to a level that the body can cope with: we do not try to ban it altogether. (See also p.114 for further information on sodium.)

We try to keep our sugar intake low so that the body is encouraged to obtain part of its energy from naturally balanced carbohydrates – the complex carbohydrates, rather than the simple carbohydrate found in refined sugar. The refining of carbohydrate has created virtual power packs of concentrated energy – in fact many products are sold on just this point – but it is really only when undertaking strenuous exercise that this sort of energy source is required. Most of us should strive to obtain our energy requirements from a mixture of complex carbohydrates, fats and protein, all of which are interchangeable as far as the body is concerned as an energy source. We should avoid as far as possible the simple carbohydrates, such as dextrose, fructose and sucrose. Carbohydrate is, of course, essential to the human brain, nerve and lung tissue, and is supplied to these areas in the form of glucose. The main problem associated with a high intake of sugars is that the excess is converted to fats (triglycerides) and stored in the body in the adipose tissue as fat. On this programme, any excess fat is bound to create a problem and overweight can lead to all sorts of complications in your condition.

We strive on the programme to lower the overall intake of fats and to guide you towards the use of less saturated fats. Fats are composed of two basic types of fatty acids: saturated (hard) and unsaturated (soft, oil-like). Natural fats are a mixture of saturated and unsaturated fatty acids. The unsaturated fatty acids are so named because of the incomplete portions of the molecule (double bonds) and may have between one and four double bonds per molecule. Those with one double bond are known as mono-unsaturated and those with two to four double bonds are known as polyunsaturated; in this latter category are the essential fatty acids (linoleic, linolenic and archidonic acid) which are required for normal health but cannot be made in the body. Enough of these fatty acids should be present in the diet to provide approximately 2% of the energy intake. The greater the number of double bonds in the fat the more soft or oil-like is its consistency and, in order to incorporate these fats in foodstuffs to give a product which has an acceptable appearance and consistency, it is necessary for manufacturers to hydrogenate them, i.e., to saturate some or all of the double bonds to give a harder fat. The prime source of unsaturated fats is fish and vegetable oils, with the major exception of coconut oil, which is classed as saturated. We should be trying also to reduce our intake of artificially-created, hydrogenated, fats. This is very convenient for the food-producer who can thus virtually dictate the shelf-life of his product, but the end product is by no means ideal for us and should be avoided as much as possible.

The reasons for a high fibre intake have been discussed in the chapter on detoxification, but I would like to add here that evidence is accumulating all the time to support the advisability of adopting a diet rich in fibre such as bran. Oat bran, for example, contains an agent called β-glucan, which carries cholesterol to the colon, and serious medical conditions such as haemorrhoids, diverticulitis, varicose veins, colitis, cancer and atherosclerosis can all be attributed in some degree to a longterm lack of consumption of fibre.

Pantothenic acid (Vitamin B_5) is essential for the proper dispersal of fats, carbohydrates and proteins. It plays a major role in the creation of amino acids, sterols and steroid hormones and it is for this main reason that it is an important ingredient of our programme. There is further information on this substance on p.98.

In our treatment programme, it is essential that we provide the body with the raw materials from which it may select its own requirements and, for this reason, it makes sense to include in our diets foods which are rich sources of nutrients. Kelp, for example, contains many, many minerals and we would do well to study which foods are good sources of some of the more obscure minerals, such as manganese. The reference section of this book discusses which foods supply which vitamins and minerals.

In the Rowland Remedy Food Guide, we have taken into account clinical observations on patients suffering with psoriasis and we have listened to the opinions of patients who have learned through trial and error which foods, food colourings and preservatives and methods of preparation have been counter-productive. The Food Guide reflects a balance of evidence for and against certain substances. Remember, however, that the essence of the self-care programme is that it is individually tailored and you will have to observe very carefully the effects of all foods and food substances on your own condition.

FUNDAMENTALS OF THE REGIME

As it is important that you should fully understand the reasons behind the diet programme, let us now look in more detail at the fundamentals of the regime; the inclusion of amino acids, an emulsifier, the 'ninety-two element diet' and the fast.

AMINO ACIDS

Amino acids are, as already mentioned, the body's basic building blocks and they are obtained from our intake of protein. There are twenty-two of them, ten of which are essential to life. These are: arginine, histidine, isoleucine, leucine, lysine, methionine, phenylalanine, threonine, tryptophan and valine.

Unlike plants, which can manufacture their own proteins, we need to obtain proteins from food and it is essential that we have a regular intake of complete proteins from such things as lean meats, fish, eggs, fowl, milk, cheese, buttermilk, yogurts, soya beans, nuts, beans, peas, yeast and grains. As the egg has a near-perfect balance of amino acids, other sources of protein are compared with it as a reference standard. Unfortunately, the kidneys may have difficulty in coping with the high albumen content of eggs, so you should restrict your egg intake to no more than three eggs a week.

Also there is the point that your amino acid intake is best obtained from a variety of sources so that thousands of different proteins can be manufactured by the body from the different amino acids broken down by the enzymes in the digestive process.

These amino acids are carried around the body by the bloodstream and are selected by the cells for use in the production of new body tissue and replacement of such important substances as antibodies, hormones, enzymes and blood cells. It is easy to see that a long-term shortage of protein creates a condition in which degenerative disease can easily set in. (It should be mentioned in passing that a very high intake of protein over a long period can be injurious to health as damage in the form of nephritis can occur. Our need for protein varies very little whether we are at work or at rest and any excess, over and above that needed for replacing the body tissue, puts a strain on the kidneys. In the stipulated diet, and following the eight-point plan for the selection of food, you should run no risk of overconsumption of protein.)

LECITHIN

The second fundamental ingredient in our diet after amino acids is a natural emulsifier called lecithin.

Most people will be aware of the danger of cholesterol deposits on the walls of the arteries. These deposits not only impede the flow of fresh, nutrient-rich blood to the cells but also become a danger to good health in themselves as the cause of heart disease. We must take steps in our diet not only to prevent the build-up of fat deposits, but also to clear away whatever fat deposits are already present in the body.

Although cholesterol is always given a bad press, I should perhaps mention that it is constantly manufactured in the body by the liver in the right amounts to utilise Vitamin D and the hormones and bile salts it requires. It is rarely this type of cholesterol, however, that gives us problems with deposits on the artery walls. The troublesome excess comes from animal fats and processed foods containing hard or saturated fats and oils which have been hydrogenated. If the body finds no use for these globules of fat, they gather together in clusters on the artery walls and become the initial cause of conditions like high blood pressure, hardened arteries, various heart diseases and strokes.

What is needed to break down these clusters is an emulsifier, a substance which acts as a sort of soap. Vegetable oils, such as sunflower and safflower, are bonded with lecithin, nature's strongest emulsifier, whose job it is to break down the globules of fat into small particles so that they are ready to be absorbed by the tissues when required.

As well as supplementing the diet with lecithin in granule form, it is wise to restrict the intake of fat to the polyunsaturated kind where lecithin is naturally present. It is interesting to note, as a bonus, that lecithin contains two important vitamins of the B complex, choline and inositol, essential to the brain, nerves, heart, lungs and in the production of certain hormones. It is also gaining a reputation as an agent that can prevent senile dementia.

THE NINETY-TWO ELEMENT DIET

The third premise on which our treatment programme is founded is that we should approach as nearly as possible a 'ninety-two element diet'. Trace elements are substances essential to plant or animal life but are present in only very small amounts. There are at least ninety-two of them and they make up the basic composition of the earth and everything in it. In that the same concentrations of salts and trace elements that make up our blood and tissues were found in the earliest seas – the primaeval soups – we can indeed be called the children of the earth. The nitrogen in the atmosphere that is 'fixed' by conversion in the soil to nitrates to feed plants is the same nitrogen that is part of the connective tissue that binds our bones together, just as the calcium in our bones is the same as the calcium that forms the rocks of our hills and mountains.

If we organise ourselves properly, then we should never be short of minerals as they are available in abundance. They are discussed in detail in the reference section on p.108, but it is worth mentioning here an obvious and balanced source of many nutrients. While we are still not sure what life is, we can at least see for ourselves the first act of growth of an embryo plant – the sprouting or germination of the seed. Although to sustain growth, it will need nutrients from water, soil and air, this initial surge of activity is supported entirely by the miniature chemical factory called the seed, in which all the natural elements are contained in the right proportions. As it is a source of balanced nutrients that we are trying to capture in our diet, it must make sense to include a high proportion of these basic forms of life; seeds, whole grains and legumes.

THE FAST

Fourthly, a 24-hour fast is part of the treatment programme. The thinking behind this is that the body needs a period in which the elimination processes may be helped, and that the kidneys can have a chance to utilise the healing and diuretic properties of grape juice over that period. The Swiss have long regarded grape juice as a way of avoiding kidney stones, and the maintenance of healthy kidneys is one of our main aims on the programme.

The easiest way to achieve a 24-hour fast is to miss the

evening meal of one day and the breakfast and midday meal of the next. The gap in eating is then spread over 2 days and no single day is spent without food.

Finally, we should look at the dietary problems created by our modern society.

FOOD COLOURS AND OTHER ADDITIVES

Today we live in a world of food preservatives, artificial emulsifiers, stabilisers, anti-oxidants, and permitted food colours. They are to be found in the recipes of most processed food products on sale today and are added for various reasons – some good, some bad.

The American Food and Drug Administration and the European Economic Community have published lists of substances which are at present considered safe to use in given quantities as food additives. They have to be listed on the label of any food product, together with the ingredients, and additives on the EEC list have the prefix 'E'. E210, for example, is benzoic acid, which is one of the additives that you must avoid whilst you are on this treatment programme.

Food Colours and Other Additives

Colours

Tartrazine	E102	yellow
Quinoline Yellow	E104	yellow/green
Yellow 2G	107	yellow
Sunset Yellow FCF	E110	yellow
Carmoisine	E122	red
Amaranth	E123	red
Ponceau 4R	E124	red
Red 2G	128	red
Patent Blue	E131	blue/violet
Indigo Carmine	E132	blue

Brilliant Blue FCF	E133	blue
Black PN	E151	black
Carbon Black	E153	black
Chocolate Brown HT	155	brown

Preservatives

Benzoic Acid	E210
Sodium Benzoate	E211
Potassium Benzoate	E212
Monosodium Glutamate	–

Numbers without an 'E' prefix are provisional.

Some of the permitted additives are known to cause allergic reactions in some people but, because they have little or no effect upon the vast majority, the product is still permitted to be sold. It is, however, difficult if not impossible, to check on the cumulative long-term effects of additives on the individual in his or her daily life and is certainly impossible to assess this before the product has been used. The reactions of Mr Average are the mainstay of the American Food and Drug Administration and the EEC.

As well as following the Rowland Remedy Food Guide, you should also exclude from your diet the food additives listed in the table above. The azo dyes have, for many years, been associated with allergic reactions, including urticaria, and their effect seems to be accentuated when combined with one of the preservatives derived from benzoic acid. Benzoic acid occurs naturally in bananas and peas and, in an extremely severe case of psoriasis, it would be as well to avoid these foods.

5 Case Histories

The programme of treatment set out in this book has had a very high success rate in controlling many hundreds of cases of psoriasis, covering the various forms of the condition described on pp.24–29. It has worked with very few exceptions for discoid psoriasis, the most common version of the disease. I am pleased to present here a few letters from clients of mine who have overcome their condition, sometimes after many long years of suffering, by using the programme. They illustrate a variety of points to bear in mind when undertaking the programme.

Our first letter is from a young man who is a member of the Asian community in the UK: psoriasis is no respecter of race, though it is more prevalent in affluent societies with their hazard-laden diets. One point of interest here is that, after the letter was written, there was a further small outbreak of the condition when dietary restrictions were lifted. When coming off the Rowland Remedy Food Guide do it slowly and study your reaction to each food as you begin to include it in your diet again.

Two years ago I started to get an itchy feeling on my skin. I put this down to some sort of allergy, but the condition became worse and my skin started to flake.

I consulted my family doctor who prescribed some cream to stop the itching but this really did not help. After trying different sorts of creams my doctor sent me to the dermatologist at the local infirmary who diagnosed the condition as psoriasis and informed me that there was no cure.

After a year of suffering I decided to visit John Rowland who had been recommended to me by a friend. I was in sheer desperation by this time, but at my first visit John convinced me that he would be able to cure me. I was immediately put on a special diet, given herbal and vitamin tablets, a specially formulated mixture and instructed on the need for a herbal bath twice a week.

Although I had to visit John for a change of prescription every six weeks I could notice the difference after the first visit. The itchy feeling started to disappear. After the second visit, the flaking started to reduce and I felt much better in myself. At about the fourth visit I could see the new skin forming and the flaking stopped completely.

Although I had to give up eating some things I liked, such as salt and sugar, I knew it was all worthwhile: I felt like a new-born person.

I remember Mr S very well: his condition was quite severe and he had tried just about everybody before coming to me. He was so delighted that my programme had worked for him that he made an appointment to see the last specialist who had been treating him to tell him the glad tidings. The reaction he received was not quite what he had bargained for; he had expected the consultant to be interested in a different approach to the problem of psoriasis, but instead he was offended that one of his patients had consulted anyone else – let alone a herbalist. The very thought was too much for his professional pride. When Mr S, a builder by trade, offered my name so that we might get our heads together on the subject, he was told, 'I'll do better than that. I'll send all my psoriasis cases to your builder's yard in future'. Happily this sort of arrogance is dying out in the medical profession and today the doctor is much more likely to pick up the phone and ask what we had used that was so successful. Mr S wrote:

I never expected, even in my wildest dreams, that so much would be achieved in such a short time. I had suffered with psoriasis for five years during which time I saw so many skin specialists that I lost count of them. I want to express my very sincere gratitude for all you have achieved for me.

One of the most rewarding cases I have treated was Andrew, a young man of 23 years old who had had the condition since the age of 10 years. One of the interesting points that he makes is how socially restricting the disease can be. You will notice, too, how Andrew fully appreciates the importance of exercise and sunlight. It should also be becoming obvious to you now that no amount of creams or ointments will do any long-term good: it always puzzles me that the intelligent people who comprise our medical profession content themselves with treating only the symptoms of a metabolic disturbance. I am always reminded of the little boy in Holland who put his finger in the dam wall . . .

At the early age of 10 I discovered after frequent visits to skin specialists that I had a condition called psoriasis. This became very embarrassing, especially as I am very keen on sport. I had to put up with looks and stares from people, so when I had to change for a football game I would wear a long vest and hide in a corner so that people wouldn't notice me. I even went home covered in mud so that I wouldn't have to shower with the others. I got very depressed as none of the creams I was given ever worked.

I was told about John Rowland about ten months ago, and within about six months the condition has completely cleared up – after all those years. I was put on a special diet and given tablets and medicines. I had to leave off white flour, sugar, salt, red meats, beer and coffee, but within two weeks it had started to clear up. I had the confidence to go out in the sun a bit as that was good for me, so things started to improve even more quickly.

The middle of the patches of psoriasis started to clear up first. First of all my stomach was clear, then my back, then my legs, and then I just had a few spots on my pelvis. I went on holiday and what few patches I had left the sun cleared up.

I can now go into a changing-room without feeling embarrassed, and I go swimming. I can wear short-sleeved shirts without people coming and saying, 'What's that there?'. My girlfriend and my family can hardly believe the change. Another benefit is that I've lost a lot of weight, and I feel much fitter.

One major point that I must make to you is the vital importance of the encouragement of other members of your family. All the family will benefit from changing to a healthier diet and the programme will help to stave off many of the degenerative diseases of our Western societies, such as arthritis, hypertension and heart disease. A recent patient of mine, Brian, owes his success in fighting a very severe case of psoriasis largely to his wife, who changed the eating habits of the whole family to make things easier for him. He was at a further disadvantage in that, as a lorry driver, he was accustomed to eat at transport cafés, many of which unfortunately still serve mostly fried food and other items which are banned from the early stages of the treatment programme. Brian's wife now fills a plastic food box with fresh fruit, wholemeal bread and an array of salads.

We felt it was important that Brian should not miss out on relaxing with other drivers, so we bent the rules a little to allow him weak tea without sugar when he visits cafés. He has also benefited enormously from losing 11kg (25lb) and he feels much fitter. The condition had been with him for over 30 years and he had been told many times that it was incurable, so to have so much relief in a matter of six months gave him a new lease of life.

The rate of success of the treatment programme is very high, but as with all things in life there are exceptions. I feel it is worthwhile examining a few cases where the programme failed. It may be that by studying these you will be able to eliminate from your life style factors which might hamper progress.

The degree of success achieved with the programme may vary with the effort put into your holistic health programme – you must be honest with yourself and recognise that you can expect only the success you deserve. Having said that, however, there have been baffling failures where I know that my clients have followed the suggested programme rigidly.

The first case of this sort that stands out in my mind was a member of a Psoriasis Association. She made great progress in the early stage of the programme but came to an abrupt halt after the second stage. There is no doubt that she tried hard but, alas, to no avail. The only reason we could think of was her age, as she was in her late 70s and had had the condition for some considerable time.

One unmarried lady schoolteacher tried the programme with great fervour, and even flew to the Dead Sea for the healing properties of the salt water, but without success.

The most recent disappointment was an exceptionally pleasant lady who stuck to the programme to the letter but with very little change at all. We thought that one possible reason for failure may have been that she was once an alcoholic and this may have had some long-term effect on the system, rendering the detoxification programme ineffectual.

Another woman, in her 30s, was unable to drink much fluid of any description (she had little more than two cups of water per day) and this could well have been the reason for failure.

I have felt it worthwhile pointing out some possible reasons for failure, but do please approach the programme with optimism. The success rate is very high indeed, and the reward of clear skin and improved general health is worth a few months of a rigid adherence to the programme.

To emphasise this point to you I am printing in full a recent letter from my post bag.

I have been a psoriasis sufferer for 15 years but am now happy to say that I am well on the way to being cured by Mr John Rowland.

Over the past 15 years I have been to umpteen Dermatologists – been admitted to many different Dermatology units for up to 4 weeks at a time. The majority of them using the same sort of treatment – creams, lotions, baths and bandages.

As anyone who suffers from the same complaint will know the treatment does help to some degree – but once back home and into a normal routine the complaint re-appears. How can anyone live a normal life covered in creams and bandages!! In utter desperation in December 1980 my parents paid for me to go to the Psoriasis Treatment Centre at the Dead Sea in Israel. I spent a week there and came home about 90% clear. Plenty of sunshine – bathing in the salty Dead Sea and a strange diet – basically nothing to eat as I couldn't eat the food. After several weeks back home it re-appeared.

For the next 4 years life carried on very much as normal – more trips to Specialists – hospitals etc. Then in October '84 I heard about John Rowland. It was through a friend who was being treated for something completely different, but who had met a psoriasis sufferer at one of his clinics.

I made an appointment to see him and made my first visit in November '84 – admittedly not very optimistic at the onset!! I was totally ignorant of herbal medicine but after listening to Mr Rowland he did seem to make sense. I had to have a complete change of diet – to take quite a lot of tablets etc, and a bathing routine.

After taking the time to see Mr Rowland I made up my mind to give the whole new way of life a fair trial. I was told the complete cure would take about 9 months. After just a couple of months an improvement was noticeable and now after six visits I am absolutely over the moon.

Admittedly it has not been easy – one has to have total commitment. It is a whole new way of life but it is great to know that you are literally curing yourself from within your own body. The routine not only cures the psoriasis but has made a new woman out of me. Several other minor ailments I suffered from have also disappeared, my whole wellbeing is greatly improved.

I am very grateful to have been given the chance to be helped by John Rowland and I sincerely hope that one day he will be recognised for his marvellous treatment by the medical profession.

Many thanks Mr Rowland.

6 The Programme

I have developed this programme of treatment for psoriasis after experience of many hundreds of clients who were suffering with the condition in its varying forms and differing degrees of severity. I have found that there are six stages of progress which one needs to go through to control the condition successfully and that at each stage the preparations used are different.

In the following pages, I outline in brief what you can hope to experience at each stage of progress. I then explain the breakfast and lunch menus, the special baths and fast periods, before explaining in detail each stage of progress and the different preparations that are used.

The ingredients of all the preparations that are recommended will be found on pp.77–81.

THE SIX STAGES OF PROGRESS

1. A feeling that you are more alive and more able to cope with your condition. You are often sleeping better.
2. The itching, if previously noticeable, starts to relent and soon becomes negligible.
3. The actual appearance of the condition becomes worse and new patches appear.
4. The crustations start to come off from the centre of the patches.
5. The skin becomes smooth with reddish areas where the psoriasis had manifested itself.
6. The skin becomes normal all over and the reddish

patches completely fade. Occasionally there is one patch of localised psoriasis left; this is often in the scalp, nails or the elbow. This area needs frequent use of the Chicko Oil or Ointment.

Your confidence that you can control your condition will now be at its height and you will be getting a little bored with the programme. This is the time for you to start to come off the strict guidelines and start to re-introduce foods into your diet one at a time, preferably at monthly intervals. In this way you will be able to tell if that food is suitable for you, particularly by the itching that precedes an area of psoriasis appearing.

If this itching appears then you should eliminate that particular food from your diet permanently. This is the way to build your own successful self-care system which is tailor-made for you.

Hopefully the Rowland Remedy Food Guide will be of great help to you during this period.

THE REGULAR MENU

BREAKFAST

Wholewheat toast and margarine
Dandelion or decaffeinated coffee

LUNCH

Salad with plenty of root vegetables and sprouting seeds
Wholewheat bread
Fresh fruit
Herbal tea
Glass of wine if desired

EVENING MEAL

The evening meal is left to your own discretion but you

must follow the general guidelines of the Rowland Remedy Food Guide as given on pp.70–76.

If you find it more convenient, it is acceptable to transpose the evening meal with the lunch menu.

BATHING

An essential part of the treatment programme is the special bath as discussed on p.39. In the early part of the programme it should be taken three times weekly. (This does not stop you having an ordinary bath on other days of the week.) Later in the programme it should be reduced to twice weekly and, later still, taken when desired. Add to the bath water ½lb (250 g) sea salt, 1 tablespoonful (20 ml) cider apple vinegar, ½ oz (15 g) chamomile flowers and 1 cupful (about 5 oz/150 g) oats.

To prepare the chamomile flowers and oats for the bath, they should be boiled for about 5 minutes. Most people find it more convenient to put them first into a muslin bag or an old stocking and then, after boiling, to add the whole contents of the plan, including the muslin bag, to the bath water, which already contains the sea salt and cider apple vinegar. The bath is now ready for your pleasure and should take about 20 or 25 minutes. Do not use soap.

If your scalp is affected then you should make an effort to immerse it in the bath water and afterwards use the shampoo described on p.81.

When you get out of the bath lightly dry yourself and apply Chicko Oil to the affected areas. Then wrap yourself up well and retire to bed where you may well perspire a little. You will be feeling in fine form at this point.

Most people derive immediate and continuous benefit from these baths without any problem.

Should you suffer from an extensive area of psoriasis, you may need to use a moisturiser, usually the one supplied by your doctor will be quite suitable, on parts of your affected areas after the bath, but only do this if you feel it is absolutely necessary.

STAGE ONE

STAGE ONE PREPARATIONS

After Breakfast

2 Multivitamin and Mineral Formula
1 Vitamin C Plus 500 mg
2 African Devil's Claw and Jamaican Sarsaparilla Compound
Dandelion Herbal Compound Tisane Drink

After Lunch

2 African Devil's Claw and Jamaican Sarsaparilla Compound
1 Vitamin C Plus 500 mg

After Evening Meal

2 African Devil's Claw and Jamaican Sarsaparilla Compound
1 Vitamin C Plus 500 mg
Dandelion Herbal Compound Tisane Drink

On Retiring

1 tablespoonful Cod Liver Oil
1 Evening Primrose Oil Capsule 500 mg

STAGE TWO

During this stage you will find an improvement in the itching if it has been present. You should be a lot more at peace with life and feeling that at last you yourself are doing something to help your own condition. It is important in any self-care system that you are in control of the treatment and we practitioners are here to help you with it when required.

During this period you should have become used to the different preparations and way of eating and should be confident enough to be trying out a more adventurous diet. There are, for example, twenty-seven varieties of beans, some sprouting, that you may eat. Also please try to include lecithin powder in your diet, possibly as a drink.

This stage may well go on for 12 weeks and you may begin to feel that you are at a standstill but this is not in fact the case.

You will note that during this stage you have added Echinacea and Periwinkle Compound to your list of preparations.

STAGE TWO PREPARATIONS

After Breakfast

2 Multivitamin and Mineral Formula
2 African Devil's Claw and Jamaican Sarsaparilla Compound
2 Echinacea and Periwinkle Compound
1 Vitamin C Plus 500 mg
Dandelion Herbal Compound Tisane Drink

After Lunch

2 African Devil's Claw and Jamaican Sarsaparilla Compound
2 Echinacea and Periwinkle Compound

After Evening Meal

2 African Devil's Claw and Jamaican Sarsaparilla Compound
1 Vitamin C Plus 500 mg
Dandelion Herbal Compound Tisane Drink

On Retiring

1 tablespoonful Cod Liver Oil
1 Evening Primrose Oil Capsule 500 mg

STAGE THREE

In Stages One and Two you will have been feeling the benefits of the vitamin, mineral and herbal preparations as well as the improved nutrition from following the food guide. This is the point at which the liver will be leading the body to complete detoxification and there may well be withdrawal symptoms and regression in your condition during this period.

Your body has been asked to do without certain food substances, such as caffeine, sugar and a high salt intake, that it may have been used to all your life. These may be the agents that your body is now craving. It is very important not to weaken in your resolve to attain good health and you should, if anything, become more vigorous in following the Rowland Remedy Food Guide.

You will also be noticing that some new patches have appeared and the crustations of the old ones are worse. The reason for this is that, in psoriasis, the whole of the skin is affected, even though it is only visible in certain areas. The new patches are the ones that had already begun to manifest themselves before you began this treatment programme and it is essential that this process continues. Thankfully this stage is shorter than the previous one and we often see the crustations starting to come away to reveal a good skin after about 9 weeks.

STAGE THREE PREPARATIONS

The preparations during Stage Three are the same as for Stage Two.

STAGE FOUR

Each stage varies in length from individual to individual and so the length of time for each of the stages is only approximate. Do not be despondent if each stage takes a little longer in your case, but rather make certain that each stage is positive before moving on to the next.

You will now be feeling that you are starting to get your reward and be more confident all round. The areas of psoriasis will be starting to clear from the centre and you should stay on the preparations but include Kelp with your Cod Liver Oil and Evening Primrose Oil.

STAGE FOUR PREPARATIONS

After Breakfast
2 Multivitamin and Mineral Formula
2 African Devil's Claw and Jamaican Sarsaparilla Compound
1 Vitamin C Plus 500 mg
Dandelion Herbal Compound Tisane Drink

After Lunch
2 African Devil's Claw and Jamaican Sarsaparilla Compound
2 Echinacea and Periwinkle Compound

After Evening Meal
2 African Devil's Claw and Jamaican Sarsaparilla Compound
2 Echinacea and Periwinkle Compound
Dandelion Herbal Compound Tisane Drink

On Retiring
1 tablespoonful Cod Liver Oil
2 Kelp Compound
1 Evening Primrose Oil Capsule 500 mg

STAGE FIVE

Your confidence that you are going to succeed in controlling your condition will grow markedly during this period as the patches of psoriasis start to disappear and the areas of skin where it had been take on a reddened appearance. There will be one or two sites still unchanged but in the main it will be much improved. You will also be a much fitter person with a normal weight. This is the bonus on any holistic programme as one always looks younger and fitter.

At this stage you should start to reduce your intake of preparations. I find that people generally find it most tiresome to remember the preparations after the midday meal, so it is probably best to discontinue these first.

STAGE FIVE PREPARATIONS

After Breakfast

2 Multivitamin and Mineral Formula
2 African Devil's Claw and Jamaican Sarsaparilla Compound
1 Vitamin C Plus 500 mg
Dandelion Herbal Compound Tisane Drink

After Lunch

No Preparations

After Evening Meal

2 African Devil's Claw and Jamaican Sarsaparilla Compound
2 Echinacea and Periwinkle Compound
Dandelion Herbal Compound Tisane Drink

On Retiring

2 Kelp Compound
1 tablespoonful Cod Liver Oil

STAGE SIX

At this point in your treatment you will have achieved a state of relative good health. The areas of skin which had been the sites of the psoriasis will have become normal and it will be difficult to see where they have been. There is often one localised spot which is left and this needs regular applications of Chicko Oil during this final stage. I find the points are found either on the elbows, scalp or nails.

You will have become bored with the programme by now and you should start to come off it. The best way to do this is to gradually relax your life style but not to slip back to your old habits of making dietary errors.

In part, the programme is educational and so you will have found out which of the foods and preparations are most suitable for you. It is now that you may become more adventurous and re-introduce one at a time some of the foods that you have been avoiding. This should be done very gradually and a diary kept, simply noting the date that you introduced the food into your diet. In this way you will be able to work out the foods that are most suitable for you.

If at any stage you begin to get that familiar itch which is the first sign of a new site of psoriasis manifesting itself then you should eliminate from your diet the last food that you have introduced on a permanent basis.

I recommend that you should take the Vitamin and Mineral Formula and the Dandelion Tisane for some time and also any of the other preparations that you felt did you most good.

This final stage will rarely be achieved in under nine months in my experience while the other stages will vary in time. Be patient and do not try to rush any stage.

STAGE SIX PREPARATIONS

After Breakfast

1 Multivitamin and Mineral Formula
2 African Devil's Claw and Jamaican Sarsaparilla Compound
Dandelion Herbal Compound Tisane Drink

ON RETIRING

Dandelion Herbal Compound Tisane Drink with any of the preparations in the programme that you felt did you the most good.

7 The Rowland Remedy Food Guide

This Food Guide is a quick reference to the foods that you may eat when on the programme. The eight-point plan has been discussed on pp.44–53, and this has been used to calculate the percentage given to each food. To recapitulate, these factors affecting the suitability of the foods are a high potassium content, a low sodium content, a low sugar content, a high pantothenic acid content, a high fibre content, that the foods should be rich sources of trace elements, and should contain no substances to which you, personally, react badly.

For Stages One to Three you may eat any foods below a 55% rating; for Stage Four any foods below 60%, and for Stages Five and Six, any foods below 70%.

When coming off the diet, the percentage can be increased by 5% per month and each addition to the diet should be studied for adverse reactions. If any present themselves then that food is not for you.

Although there is no control on the quantity of any food consumed, there are borderline foods which may rate just under your percentage. You must not have too many of these in your overall diet: it should be well-balanced. Also remember that I have not taken into account the food additives and colours. These are listed on pp. 52–53 and it is up to you to check the ingredients of each foodstuff.

FOOD VALUES

%	
	Almonds
15	dried
75	roasted, salted
15	Apple, raw, unpeeled
50	Apple juice, bottled
80	Apple sauce, sweetened
	Apricots
70	canned
20	dried
75	cooked, sweetened
15	fresh
75	nectar, concentrated
	Asparagus
75	canned
40	frozen spears, cooked
40	green, cooked
40	low sodium
	Aubergine/Egg plant,
20	cooked
30	Avocado pear
70	Bacon
95	Baking powder/soda
15	Banana
15	Barley, pearled, light
15	Bass, sea
	Beans
50	canned
15	cooked
5	mung
5	sprouts
	Beef
95	hamburger
90	canned roast
85	corned
85	dried
	lean (grilled, roasted,
75	braised)
90	pie, commercial
75	pie, homemade
	stew, canned with
85	vegetables
75	stew, homemade

%	
	Beet/beetroot
65	canned, regular pack
50	cooked
40	low sodium
60	Beet greens, cooked
	Beverages, alcoholic
80	bitter beer
30	lager beer
40	mild beer
85	gin
10	table wine
15	Blackberries
20	Blueberries
70	Bouillon cube
	Bran with sugar and
75	malt extract
50	Bran flakes (40% bran)
50	with raisins
10	Brazil nuts
	Breads
20	cracked wheat
60	French or Vienna
10	rye, American
5	pumpernickel
	white 3-4% nonfat
80	milk solids
20	wholemeal
10	wholewheat
10	Broccoli spears
10	Brussel sprouts
	Butter
85	salted
55	unsalted
10	Buttermilk
20	Cabbage, cooked
80	Cakes, (home recipe)
85	angel food
85	chocolate with icing
45	fruit, dark
45	gingerbread
45	plain without icing
75	sponge

%	
5	Carrots
80	canned, regular pack
45	cooked
60	low sodium
5	Cashew nuts, unsalted
	Cauliflower
30	cooked
5	fresh
10	frozen, cooked
	Celery
10	cooked
5	fresh
80	Chard, Swiss, cooked
	Cheese, half fat
50	Caerphilly
50	Cheddar
50	Cheshire
70	cottage
70	cream
50	Danish blue
50	Edam
50	Gruyère (Swiss)
20	Parmesan
80	Cheese, any full fat
10	Cherries
90	canned, syrup pack
50	frozen
10	Chicken
10	Chicory
	Chilli con carne,
50	canned with beans
	Chilli powder with
50	seasonings
85	Chocolate, bitter
	Clams
45	canned
	hard, round, meat
35	only
30	raw, soft meat only
	Coconut
75	dried, sweetened
50	fresh, shredded
	Coffee
20	decaffeinated
85	instant dry powder
	Corn
90	rice and wheat flakes
95	shredded
90	puffed
	Corn, sweet
	canned, whole kernel
75	regular pack
55	cooked
55	low sodium pack
85	Cornflakes
85	sugar-coated
	Cornmeal/polenta or
70	maize meal
	Cowpeas
70	canned, regular pack
40	dry seeds, cooked
60	immature, cooked
35	Crabmeat, canned
	Crackers
75	plain
75	soda
40	wholewheat
	Cranberry
45	juice
45	sauce
	Cream
85	half and half
90	light coffee
	substitute (cream, skim
95	milk, lactose)
95	whipping–light
60	Cucumbers, not peeled
75	Custard, baked
	Dandelion
10	coffee
10	greens, cooked
15	Dates
75	Doughnuts, cake-type
15	Duck, flesh only
	Eggs
60	white
	whole (no more than 3
60	per week)
60	yolk
45	Endive, curly
10	Fats, vegetable

%	
	Figs
20	canned
20	dried, uncooked
15	fresh
20	Flounder
	Fruit cocktail
20	fresh
	Gelatine
70	dry
75	sweetened, ready to eat
10	Goose, flesh only
	Grapefruit
85	canned, sweetened
75	fresh
75	juice
20	Grapes
75	juice, bottled
	Haddock
	fried (dipped in egg,
60	milk, breadcrumbs)
15	raw
	Heart, beef
80	cooked, braised
75	lean
15	Herb teas
20	Herring
	Honey (1 teaspoonful daily only at the start of your programme – no reasonable limit when you have reached
55	70 in your programme)
	Ice cream, no added salt
60	approximately 12% fat
80	Jams and preserves
80	Jellies
	Kale cooked, leaves
10	with stems
	Lamb, average of lean
75	cuts, cooked
85	Lard

%	
	Lemon juice, fresh
50	(1 daily only)
80	Lemonade, frozen, diluted
20	Lettuce
75	Lime juice, fresh or canned
75	Limeade, frozen, diluted
	Liver, cooked, fried
65	beef
65	calf
55	pork
25	Lobster, canned or cooked
25	Macaroni
70	with cheese, baked
	Margarine
75	salted
20	unsalted
	Milk
20	dry, nonfat, instant
80	evaporated, undiluted
10	goat's
20	skimmed
80	whole pasteurised
85	Milk beverages
	chocolate flavoured
80	with skimmed milk
80	malted with whole milk
30	Mineral water
10	Molasses
	Mushrooms
70	canned
10	fresh
	Mustard, prepared
65	yellow
50	Mustard greens, cooked
20	Nectarine
50	Noodles
10	Oatmeal
60	cooked, salted
10	Oil, vegetable
10	Okra, cooked
	Olives
75	green
60	ripe

%	
	Onion
15	cooked
10	fresh
	Orange
70	juice
70	peeled
10	Oyster
20	Papaya, raw
20	Parsley
20	Parsnips, cooked
	Peach
55	canned
85	cooked with sugar
	dried, sulphured,
25	uncooked
10	fresh
50	frozen
85	nectar
80	Peanut butter
	Peanuts
50	roasted
80	salted
	Pear
30	canned
10	fresh
95	nectar
	Peas
50	canned, regular pack
30	dry, split
30	frozen
10	green, cooked
20	low sodium pack
10	Pecans
	Pepper, sweet, green
10	raw
10	Perch, ocean, Atlantic
10	Persimmon, Japanese
75	Pickles
	Pies, home recipes,
	wholewheat flour
75	apple
75	cherry
75	custard
90	lemon meringue
90	mince
70	pumpkin

%	
70	Piecrust, baked
50	Pike, walleye
	Pineapple
20	canned, unsweetened
10	fresh
	juice, canned
10	unsweetened
	Pizza, cheese, home
60	recipe
	Plums
10	canned, purple
10	fresh
90	Popcorn, salted
	Pork
70	fresh, lean, roasted
70	Picnic ham, lean, simmered
	Pork, cured
80	canned, spiced or unspiced
	ham, lightcure, lean
70	cooked
	Potatoes
10	baked
10	boiled, unsalted
90	French fried
60	mashed with milk
	potato chips, using
75	vegetable oil
80	Pretzels
	Prunes
20	cooked without sugar
20	dried, uncooked
20	juice
85	Pudding, home recipe
85	bread with raisins
85	chocolate
85	cornstarch (blancmange)
85	rennin, using mix
85	rice with raisins
85	tapioca cream
	Pumpkin, canned
30	unsalted
20	Radishes
20	Raisins
70	Raspberries
75	Relish (chutney)
	Rhubarb, cooked,

%	
90	unsweetened
20	Rice
	Rice cereals
70	flakes
50	puffed, without salt
	Rolls
70	commercial, plain
70	sweet
50	wholewheat
30	Rye flour, light
70	Rye wafers
	Salad dressings
	commercial mayonnaise
75	type
75	French
60	home-cooked
65	mayonnaise
65	Thousand Island
10	Salmon, pink
55	canned
	Sardines, Pacific, canned
50	in tomato sauce
55	Sauerkraut
75	Sausage
75	Bologna
65	Frankfurters, raw
70	pork links, cooked
55	Scallops, bay, steamed
50	Shrimps, fresh
80	Sorbet/sherbert, orange
	Soup, canned, diluted
	with equal part water
50	bean
70	bean with pork
75	beef bouillon
75	beef noodle
50	chicken
	clam chowder, Manhattan
50	type
50	cream soup (mushroom)
50	lentil
50	minestrone
50	onion
50	pea, green
70	tomato
80	vegetable with beef broth
20	Spaghetti
70	home recipe
	in tomato sauce with
70	cheese
	with tender meatballs,
80	canned
	Spinach
50	canned, regular pack
15	cooked
10	fresh
40	low sodium
	Squash
20	summer, cooked
10	winter, cooked
	Strawberries
75	fresh
75	frozen
	Sugar
85	brown
85	granulated
	Sweet potatoes
15	baked
75	boiled, candied
85	Syrup, table blend
	Tangerines
70	fresh
75	juice, canned
10	Tapioca
75	Tea
15	herb
	Tomatoes
75	canned, low sodium
75	canned, regular pack
70	fresh
	juice, canned, regular
85	pack
	ketchup, regular
85	pack
80	Tongue, beef, braised
	Tuna, canned in oil,
55	solids and liquids
	Turkey
15	dark
10	light
	Turnip
20	cooked, diced

%	
30	frozen
	greens, canned, regular
40	pack
10	Vinegar, cider
85	Waffles, home recipe
10	Walnuts
20	Watermelon
-	Wheat and malted
55	barley, dry, cooked
30	Wheat, rolled, cooked
10	Wheatbran, crude
	Wheat cereals
55	cooked
65	flakes
10	puffed, without salt
10	shredded, plain
	Wheatflours
55	all-purpose or family cake
55	self-raising
10	wheatgerm
10	wholewheat
55	White sauce
10	Yeast, baker's
	Yogurt, made from partially
10	skimmed milk

8 JR Preparations Guide

RR405 Kelp Tablets

Seaweeds were the first living plants on the earth and there are over 700 recorded species now in existence. There is good reason to believe that kelp is one of the first crops to have been used by Man. It was certainly used by the Chinese, the Greeks and the Romans not only as a food, but also as a fertiliser and as a medicine. In Ireland, Wales and Japan, seaweed is a common food today.

I have found kelp to be beneficial in the treatment of both over- and underactive thyroid glands, which suggests a complex make-up of nutrients. I have mentioned earlier that our blood mimics, and therefore resembles very closely, the chemical consistency of sea water. Kelp, in absorbing the nutrients of sea water and processing them into a form that humans can use has done a good job for us. You will not be surprised that kelp tablets are included as a supplement in your total health programme. An average analysis of kelp shows that it contains thirteen vitamins, sixty trace elements and twenty essential amino acids. Please note, particularly if you are a vegetarian, that kelp contains Vitamin B_{12}, an ingredient that is often deficient in the vegetarian diet.

RR407 JR Multivitamin and Mineral Formula

Although you will not be deficient in very many vitamins and minerals at any one time, by taking this formula

regularly you will ensure that you lack none of the vital ingredients for making as speedy as possible a recovery. You should take 2 tablets daily with food.
Each tablet will provide:

VITAMINS	
Vitamin A (retinol)★	500 μg(1450 i.u.)
Vitamin D_3 (cholecalciferol)	4 μg(160 i.u.)
Vitamin E (dl–α tocopheryl acetate)	10 mg(10 i.u.)
Vitamin C (ascorbic acid)	50 mg
Vitamin B_1 (thiamine HCl)	20 mg
Vitamin B_2 (riboflavin)	20 mg
Vitamin B_6 (pyridoxine HCl)	20 mg
Vitamin B_{12} (cyanocobalamin)	4 μg
Nicotinamide	20 μg
Pantothenic acid	20 mg
d-Biotin	150 mg
Folic acid	200 μg
Para-aminobenzoic acid	10 mg
Choline bitartrate	10 mg
Inositol	5 mg
MINERALS	
Calcium (as phosphate)	126 mg
Phosphorus (as phosphate)	60 mg
Potassium (as phosphate)	20 mg
Magnesium (as oxide)	25 mg
Iron (as ferrous fumarate)	3 mg
Copper (as gluconate)	100 μg
Manganese (as gluconate)	2.2 mg
Iodine (as kelp)	20 μg
Zinc (as oxide)	1 mg
Selenium (as Se yeast)	25 μg

★1 μg = 2.907 international units (i.u)

Other ingredients

Lecithin	20 mg
Betaine HCl	2.2 mg
dl-Methionine	2.2 mg
l-Lysine HCl	1.75 mg
cl-Cysteine HCl	0.25 mg
Glutamic acid	4 mg
Bioflavonoids complex	5 mg
Dried yeast	20 mg
Alfalfa	20 mg
Kelp	25 mg
Ginseng	20 mg
Red Clover	5 mg
Damiana	3 mg

RR 410 Aly Salt

Aly Salt is potassium chloride It is an alternative to common sodium chloride, common table salt. It should be used on the food after cooking and not in the original food preparation.

RR 411 Vitamin C Plus

These tablets each contain 500 mg of ascorbic acid with the addition of 50 mg of the bioflavonoid complex.

RR 412 African Devil's Claw and Jamaican Sarsaparilla Compound

The ingredients are African devil's claw (*Harpogophytum procumbens*) and Sarsaparilla (*Smilax ornata*).

RR 413 Echinacea and Periwinkle Compound

The ingredients are echinacea (*Echinacea angustifolia*) and periwinkle (*Vinca major*).

RR 414 Dandelion Herbal Compound Tisane

Yellow dock *Rumex crispus*
Burdock *Arctium lappa*
Wood sanicle *Sanicula europaea*
Buchu *Barosma betulina*
Sarsaparilla (Jamaican) *Smilax ornata*
Skullcap *Scutellaria Laterifolia*
Dandelion *Taraxacum officinale*
Red clover *Trifolium pratense*

DIRECTIONS FOR USE

1. Place 2 teaspoonsful in a small teapot.
2. Pour on ½ pint (300 ml) boiling water and stir.
3. Leave to stand overnight.
4. Strain. Take 1 cupful after breakfast and evening meal.

RR 418 Cod Liver Oil Capsules

People often prefer to take capsules of cod liver oil rather than the oil itself. This is acceptable in the programme.

RR420 Chicko Oil

The Chicko Oil formula has benefited a great many of my patients. It is a blend of vegetable oils that combine to help the skin back into good health. It should be used frequently on localised areas and after the special baths.

Where the cover of psoriasis is extensive you may well need a moisturiser as well. The moisturiser has often been supplied by the doctor and this is quite adequate for the job. If this is necessary, select one area of the body upon which to use the Chicko Oil regularly and use the moisturiser on the rest. As your condition improves, extend the use of the Chicko Oil all over the body to get the full benefit of its healing properties.

The ingredients are chickweed oil (*Stellaria media*), olive oil (*Olea europaea*) and almond oil (*Prunus communis*).

RR 422 Evening Primrose Oil Capsules

Evening primrose oil is yet another example of how the herbalist has contributed to modern medicine. The oil, which is pressed from the seeds, is beneficial not only to people who have skin problems but also in reducing the build-up of cholesterol in arteries and reversing liver damage in alcoholics.

It is now gaining considerable support in hospitals throughout the world, where it is being prescribed for pre-menstrual tension, heart disease and vascular problems.

The plant is a native of Mexico but is being cultivated in large quantities in Europe.

RR 423 Herbal Psoriasis Shampoo

A traditional shampoo, this contains herbs and nutrients known to benefit those on an holistic programme. Two of the main constituents are chickweed and chamomile.

Part 3
Reference Section

9 Herbal Compendium

African devil's claw	*Harpogophytum procumbens*
Alfalfa	*Medicago*
Almond	*Prunus communis*
Buchu	*Barosma betulina*
Burdock	*Arctium lappa*
Chamomile	*Matricaria chamomilla*
Chickweed	*Stellaria media*
Damiana	*Turnera aphrodisiaca*
Dandelion	*Taraxacum officinale*
Ginseng	*Acanthopanax senticosus maxim*
Kelp	*Laminaria* spp.
Olive	*Olea europaea*
Periwinkle	*Vinca major*
Red clover	*Trifolium pratense*
Sarsaparilla	*Smilax ornata*
Skullcap	*Scutellaria laterifolia*
Wood sanicle	*Sanicula europaea*

African Devil's Claw *Harpogophytum procumbens*

Constituents: Iridoid, glycosides.
Action: Anti-inflammatory, astringent, bitters.

One of nature's greatest assets is its ability to restore itself if left alone by Man or its natural predator, fire.

A plant can become apparently extinct and, two or three generations later, reappear from seeds that have been dormant in the soil just waiting to be stimulated into action by some force or other.

Just such a thing happened to devil's claw. The plant which was one of the main herbs in the witch doctor's dispensary in southern Africa seemed to become extinct around the turn of the century, probably due to overuse: it is the secondary tubers which are used for their medicinal qualities and these are the plant's store of food.

In the early 1960s there was flooding in the part of Africa which used to grow devil's claw and shortly after this the plant made a resurgence of growth, much to the delight of the natives of the region, some of whom had only heard of the plant by the many tales which had been handed down as part of the folklore.

Some of these tales were quite harrowing as many of their forebears had perished in the desert because of this plant. It grows in semi-desert regions and looks a little like a starfish close to the ground: at dusk it is difficult to see. If you were to step on the centre of the plant the tentacles would react and grip your foot so tightly that you would be unable to prise the plant open again. I imagine that this would be the basis for many folk tales about gruesome deaths, and it explains also the name of devil's claw which was given it by the natives.

Alfalfa *Medicago*

Constituents: Source of vitamins, mineral salts, potassium, phosphorus, iron.

Action: Nutritive.

Alfalfa is a rich source of nutrients, particularly potassium, phosphorus, and iron, which are obtained by the roots of the plant which extend deep into the ground, sometimes as much as 40 feet (12 m). It has recently become a popular food supplement for people on fitness programmes and those who are convalescing.

Almond *Prunus communis*

Constituents: Fixed oil, consisting mainly of olein and a small proportion of linolein.

Action: Nutritive and demulcent.

Most people will be familiar with the almond nut, if not the oil, but we use both at some stage of the programme. The oil is one of the ingredients in Chicko Oil which is used for the massage after the special baths and the nut will be found in the muesli.

The almond tree is mainly found in warm climates but it has always been popular in gardens in temperate climates.

The nutritive value of the nut has made it popular with naturopaths who frequently recommend that ten almonds be taken daily, chewed well.

Buchu *Barosma betulina*

Constituents: Volatile oil and an agent called diosphenol which has antiseptic qualities.

Action: Urinary antiseptic, diuretic, diaphoretic, anti-inflammatory.

I have found the beneficial effects of this herb to be tremendous; it has undoubted powers as a urinary antiseptic and I have achieved remarkable results by basing a formula on buchu for such conditions as cystitis, gravel and inflammation of the bladder, as well as arthritis. In fact, I had an enquiry from one of Britain's leading hospitals asking how I had successfully treated a patient of theirs with whom they had had little success. I explained that I was using a herb that was first introduced into medicine in this country in 1821 and was, for over a hundred years, the official treatment for cystitis, urethritis and catarrh of the bladder. With the advent of antibiotics it lost its popularity but not its usefulness; it is as good today as it was in 1821.

Burdock *Arctium lappa*

Constituents: Inulin, bitters, resin, fixed and volatile oils, flavonoids, anti-bacterial substances.

Action: Mild diuretic, anti-bacterial, alterative.

Burdock was used by the herbalists in their treatment for gonorrhea before the advent of antibiotics. It has always been regarded as a strong alterative or blood cleanser and is today used in treatments for arthritis, gout, eczema and psoriasis and is often used in conjunction with slippery elm bark in treating anorexia nervosa.

Apart from its contribution to herbal medicine, burdock has two other claims to fame: the first one is the burrs which are the plant's means of disseminating itself, hence the various synonyms by which it is referred to throughout the world such as thorny burr, beggar's buttons or hoppy major. It is also one of the basic ingredients of that popular drink, dandelion and burdock.

Chamomile (German) *Matricaria chamomilla*

Constituents: Volatile oil, anthemic and tannic acids.

Action: Tonic, carminative, stomachic.

The German Chamomile is easily distinguished by its white flower head which is about 20 mm (1 in) in diameter. These are the heads to be used in the special baths for the most successful treatments. If these are not available then one of the other varieties of chamomile should be used but at double the quantity.

There are numerous varieties of chamomile, some of which can be found in most countries of the world. This is due in part to its reputation as a medicinal herb and to a large part its popularity as a garden plant.

It was also popular in the past with the Egyptians who revered it for its virtues and dedicated it to their gods.

The countryfolk in Lancashire still regard chamomile as

one of their greatest herbal remedies, even for their animals. Only this year a farmer came to me and bought out my entire stock of the herb so that he could feed it to one of his cows that was off colour. He reported to me a few days later that the cow was well again. Chamomile tea is becoming a very popular way of taking the benefits of the herb and there are an increasing number of firms throughout the world who are now selling it as an alternative to ordinary tea. If you have not yet tried it please do, and you will be pleasantly surprised.

Chickweed *Stellaria media*

Constituents: Saponins.

Action: Anti-rheumatic, alterative, antiseptic, demulcent.

Chickweed spread around the world at about the same rate that the world became Westernised, and so will be familiar to most people reading this book. It has been used in herbal medicine for internal preparations and for Chickweed Ointment which is useful for conditions of the skin, particularly psoriasis. This is the reason why chickweed is one of the major ingredients of Chicko Oil.

I remember that another well known Lancashire herbalist, A. Hool, wrote a book on his herbal remedies and much of it was devoted to chickweed which had until then been little used by herbalists outside Lancashire.

Damiana *Turnera aphrodisiaca*

Constituents: Volatile oils, bitters, resins and tannins.

Action: Tonic reputed to act directly on the reproductive organs.

Damiana is a native of South America and Mexico where it gained a high and justifiable reputation as a tonic which acts directly on the reproductive organs. There is no doubt in my opinion that it has beneficial results in helping the body restore itself to good health, which is why I often include the herb in my formulas.

The herb is still popular in the folk medicine of Mexico and Brazil where the various methods of preparing the herb for use are still handed down from father to son.

Dandelion *Taraxacum officinale*

Constituents: Bitters, taraxacerin, glycosides, potassium.
Action: Anti-rheumatic, diuretic, anti-inflammatory, mild laxative.

The dandelion is a familiar plant to us all and a particularly useful one, both for its edible and medicinal properties. It gets its name from a corruption of the French name 'dent de lion' because the leaves have a jagged appearance that resembles the teeth of lions.

The leaves are used in salads and they have a slightly bitter taste when young. They are often used boiled as a substitute for spring cabbage or spinach. The plant is popular as a partner in that famous drink dandelion and burdock. The roots are roasted to form dandelion coffee – a very pleasant drink which I recommend as an excellent substitute for tea or ordinary coffee. The absence of caffeine is a bonus to anyone on a detoxification programme.

The history of dandelion as a medicinal plant goes back hundreds if not thousands of years. There are many early references in India to dandelions being most suitable for liver complaints. This is probably because the root contains a bitter substance called taraxacerin which is active against diseases of the liver.

It is also beneficial to the kidney and urinary systems and is a general stimulant to the system.

Apart from its uses in compounds for arthritis, herbalists would use it for such conditions as cholecystitis, gall stones and jaundice.

Ginseng *Acanthopanax senticosus maxim*

Constituents: Glycosides, eleutherocides.

Action: Tonic.

There are many different varieties of ginseng to be found in many different parts of the world but few of them have scientific data published on them to the same level as this one.

It has been shown to have an invigorating effect on Man, increasing his physical and mental capacities and strengthening his resilience to stress and fatigue. Because of this it has been administered to astronauts and cosmonauts to improve their performance.

Ginseng grows wild in many places throughout the world but is found in abundance in China, Russia and Korea. It is sometimes called Russian Root, Eleutherococcus or Panax.

As with all ginsengs the best results are obtained from the roots of shrubs which are between six and seven years old. These will contain the right glycosides, vitamins and minerals to help our bodies attain the good health we are seeking.

Vitamins E, B_1, B_6, B_{15}, and B_{12} have been shown to exist in the root, so it is an especially good herb to include in a vegetarian diet.

Kelp *Laminaria* spp.

Constituents: A wide range of minerals and trace elements, the most important being iodine.

Action: Protects against infection, regulates and activates metabolism.

See pp.77 for details of this substance.

Olive *Olea europaea*

Constituents: Oil, resin.

Action: Antiseptic, astringent, febrifuge, demulcent, mild laxative.

My chief interest in olive is the use of the oil in Chicko Oil and for taking internally, combined with lemon juice, as a tonic to the liver.

You will undoubtedly be familiar with olive oil, but perhaps not aware of the process which is used for extraction. The first pressing of the fruit is achieved by crushing the olives in rough bags which are immersed in water. The oil which floats on the water is skimmed off and this oil has a slight green tint and is referred to as 'virgin' or 'first pressing'. This is available in most good shops and is the one that we want for our programme.

To obtain the second pressing of the oil, the cake is moistened and allowed to ferment: this is not the quality for us.

Periwinkle *Vinca major*

Constituents: Alkaloids, glycosides, bitters.
Action: Astringent, tonic, anti-inflammatory, alterative.

There are three main varieties of periwinkle to be found in most countries of the world and they have all been used in herbal medicine for many generations. The *Vinca major* which is the variety I use with Echinacea has long had the reputation for curing a type of diabetes. Trials for its efficacy in this direction were dropped when Banting and Best made their discovery of insulin.

On further trials to see if it would be helpful in controlling cancer the Madagascar periwinkle was shown to have a number of alkaloids, two of which are today in regular use in our hospitals combating leukaemia.

The complex nature of the plant makes it the ideal aid in the detoxification process which I have described as part of the holistic treatment programme.

Red Clover *Trifolium pratense*

Constituents: Glycosides.
Action: Dermatological agents.

The use of red clover for psoriasis and eczema is taken so much for granted by traditional herbalists as it has been used as one of our standard alteratives for generations.

It has also featured as one of the most successful agents that we have in combating various forms of cancer, particularly when combined with violet leaves and red beetroot, and this has given red clover its popularity.

It is also very efficient in the detoxification programme for psoriasis, and its alterative powers are a major contribution to the success of the Dandelion Herbal Compound Tisane drink.

Sarsaparilla (Jamaican) *Smilax ornata*

Constituents: Saponins, glycosides.
Action: Anti-rheumatic, antiseptic, alterative.

Sarsaparilla is famous as a drink which is often sold alongside dandelion and burdock, each having their own distinct flavour. It is one of the strongest alteratives that we have and its powers for cleansing the blood and giving a clear skin are renowned.

It was first introduced into the UK in the sixteenth century for the treatment of syphilis and other venereal diseases, and in all probability will soon be required again as antibiotics are now starting to be non-effective in this area of disease. More recently it has been used for other chronic conditions, such as arthritis, where it is still popular to this day in herbal medicine.

Skullcap *Scutellaria laterifolia*

Constituents: Flavonoid glycosides, volatile oil, tannin,

bitters.
Action: Sedative, anti-spasmodic.

Before stronger synthetic sedatives came onto the market, skullcap was considered to be almost a specific for the convulsive twitchings of St Vitus' Dance.

It still has a tremendous following amongst insomniacs as a pleasant way of inducing sleep without any of the unpleasant side effects of synthetic drugs.

The anti-spasmodic effect of skullcap has ensured its place in the folklore of Europe and the USA for its ability to cure hiccups.

Wood Sanicle *Sanicula europaea*

Constituents: Tannin, bitters.
Action: Astringent, alterative, anti-inflammatory.

The origin of the name sanicle is the Latin word 'sano', 'heal or cure'.

In the Middle Ages, it gained a high reputation for treating conditions of the blood, being said to cleanse the body of morbid material, leaving the blood healthier and in better condition. This is just right for the psoriasis programme where detoxification is the main theme.

It is often combined with other herbs rather than used on its own.

Glossary

Alkaloid	Nitrogenous compound found in living plants and containing their active principle, e.g. quinine or caffeine.
Alterative	Helps cleanse the system of morbid matter.
Anti-bacterial	Improves body defence against infection.

Anti-bilious	Corrects the bile.
Anti-inflammatory	Reduces inflammation.
Anti-rheumatic	Relieves rheumatic and arthritic conditions.
Antiseptic	Destroys micro-organisms, prevents sepsis.
Anti-spasmodic	Relieves or prevents spasms.
Astringent	Counteracts excessive body secretions.
Carminative	Expels wind.
Demulcent	Lubricative.
Diaphoretic	Stimulates perspiration.
Diuretic	Increases the formation and discharge of urine.
Febrifuge	Dispelling fever.
Glycoside	Any group of organic compounds found abundantly in plants which hydrolyse into sugar and other organic compounds.
Laxative	Mild purgative.
Nutritive	Nourishing.
Resin	A semi-solid substance obtained from exudations of plants.
Saponins	Glycosides found in plants which cause water to froth.
Sedative	Soothing to the nerves.
Stomachic	Strengthens stomach and digestive organs.
Tannin	Astringent vegetable compounds.
Tonic	Assists in strengthening the system.
Volatile oil	Odiferous oil obtained from plants containing a variety of chemical compounds.

10 Vitamins

Here we look at the vitamins with which you are likely to come into contact when on a treatment programme. For each of the vitamins current to date, I have outlined the relevant data, function, natural sources and deficiency manifestations. I have also made a personal comment as to the attention you need to pay to ensure you have an adequate supply of each vitamin.

Vitamins are a group of substances essential to life which are found in foodstuffs. They are potent organic compounds, although they are found only in very small concentrations. For a substance to be classified as a vitamin, it must firstly perform specific functions in the cells and body tissues; secondly, the body must be unable to synthesise sufficient for its needs; and thirdly, its absence would result in a deficiency disease.

An important point which you should understand is that vitamins found in nature work synergistically, that is, they work together creating a greater force than the sum of their parts. This co-operation is found in many areas, but one very notable synergistic action is that of the B complex vitamins. Thus, although it is acceptable to take a single Vitamin B factor as a supplement it is necessary to ensure that your intake of the whole B complex is adequate.

Vitamin A

Fat soluble.
Measured in micrograms (μg).

Retinol is Vitamin A.
Carotene precursor is converted to Vitamin A at a ratio of 6:1.
Works in conjunction with Vitamin D.

Functions: maintains healthy epithelial cells, mucous membranes, skin and bone.

Natural sources: liver, egg yolk, dairy produce, vegetables, apricots, cod liver oil.

Deficiency manifestations: dry mucous membranes, loss of taste and smell, rough or dry skin, glare or night blindness.

Note: an important vitamin, especially for the health of the eye. It is as well to pay particular attention to your intake of this vitamin if you are a smoker, or watch a lot of television or if you spend a lot of time under fluorescent light.

The fact that this vitamin is fat-soluble means that it can build up in the liver and, if too much is taken, Vitamin A toxicity can result.

You obtain Vitamin A direct from foods as retinol, or from the substance called carotene which the body converts to Vitamin A.

Vitamin B_1 Thiamine

Water-soluble, thus excess is excreted by body and regular intake required.
Measured in milligrams (mg).
Tissues of the heart, liver, brain and kidneys have the highest concentrations in the body.

Functions: essential for growth. Aids digestion and the conversion of carbohydrates into energy. Improves confidence. Aids the muscles and nerves, particularly the heart muscles, in functioning correctly.

Natural sources: wheatgerm, nuts, beans, whole grains, pulses, dairy foods.

Deficiency manifestations: nervous disorders, irritability, brain fag, easy exhaustion, poor digestion, depressed state.

Note: you may recall reading in your history books about the disease beri beri, caused by a severe deficiency of Vitamin B. Until the discovery of the cause of the condition by Dr Edward Vedder in the Philippines in 1910, this disease was responsible for many deaths. Dr Vedder cured babies dying of beri beri by giving them rice bran.

The subsequent discovery of the Vitamin B_1 was made by Dr R.R. Williams and from this discovery stemmed the ability to synthesise the vitamin. This largely eradicated the disease. It should be re-emphasised, however, how important bran or fibre can be in our diets.

If you are a smoker or a drinker then you will almost certainly need plenty of thiamine. People who have a high sugar intake may also be at risk of a deficiency.

Vitamin B_2 Riboflavin

Water-soluble and, though the body storage is slightly better than thiamine, a daily intake is still indicated.

Measured in milligrams (mg)

Stable to heat, acid and oxidation.

Sensitive to alkali.

Should be stored in the dark as it is destroyed by light when in solution.

Functions: essential to a number of chemical reactions in the body for the release of energy within the cell, thus growth, and for healthy skin, gums and eyes.

Natural sources: wheatgerm, liver, soya beans, eggs, vegetables, milk, cheese, fish.

Deficiency manifestations: nervousness, irritability, dry hair, dry skin, mouth ulcers, ocular problems such as frontal headaches, eye strain, itching and sensitivity to light.

Note: riboflavin functions as part of a group of enzymes called flavoproteins which are vital to the metabolism of carbohydrates, fats and proteins. It also has an important role to play in the health of the eye.

Vitamin B_3 Niacin

Water soluble.

Measured in milligrams (mg).

Stable in dry state, even in alkali.

Comes in two forms: nicotinic acid and nicotinamide.

Functions: involved in the synthesis of proteins and fats, therefore helpful to healthy skin, the gastro-intestinal tract and nervous system. Helps reduce cholesterol deposits.

Natural sources: liver, lean meats, whole grains, fish, eggs, nuts, dates, prunes.

Deficiency manifestations: pellagra, a disease which affects the skin, digestive system and nervous system.

Note: niacin, nicotinic acid and nicotinamide have nothing at all to do with nicotine as found in tobacco.

The body's requirements are uncertain, though it seems to obtain its supplies by converting the amino acid tryptophan into niacin. This process requires the presence of pyridoxine (Vitamin B_6), an example of the need to ensure the presence of all the B Vitamins.

Vitamin B_5 Pantothenic Acid

Water soluble.

Measured in milligrams (mg).

Functions: part of a co-enzyme which plays a role in the metabolism of carbohydrates, fats and proteins, allowing the release of energy. Aids in the synthesis of amino acids, the body's basic building blocks, fatty acids, sterols, and steroid hormones. Essential to the formation of porphyrin, the pigment portion of the haemoglobin molecule.

Natural sources: liver, kidney, heart, wholewheat bread, brown rice, salmon, eggs, nuts, broccoli.

Deficiency manifestations: hair loss, grey hair, dry skin, digestive disorders.

Note: the word 'pantothenic' means widespread, which gives you some idea of the importance put on this vitamin by nature.

Pantothenic acid plays a vital role in the programme of treatment because of its function in aiding the synthesis of amino acids, the sterols and the body's own steroid hormones which are essential for the body to be able to heal itself.

A high pantothenic acid content is one of the factors in the eight-point Rowland Remedy Food Guide.

Vitamin B_6 Pyridoxine

Water soluble and regular supply needed due to poor retention by the body.
Measured in milligrams (mg).
Stable to light and oxidation.
Considerable losses occur in refining, or in heating food above boiling point.

Functions: essential for healthy muscle, skin and nerves. Enables the body to use protein more efficiently, also to convert tryptophan to niacin.

Natural sources: glandular meats, lamb, legumes, potatoes, oats, wheatgerm, bananas. Some may be found in vegetables such as cabbage and carrot.

Deficiency manifestations: muscle cramps, anaemia, irritability, depression. In cases of severe shortage, the onset of convulsions and formation of kidney stones may present.

Note: I have prescribed pyridoxine over a long period for problems associated with the menopause, particularly the depressive state. The most successful dose seems to be 300 mg daily.

A regular dose of 100 mg daily, throughout the cycle, is sufficient for other disorders, such as pre-menstrual syndrome, and I recommend between 50 mg and 100 mg regularly if oral contraceptives are being used.

Vitamin B_{12} Cyanocobalamin (Cobalamin)

Water soluble.
Measured in micrograms (μg).
Stable during cooking.

Functions: A co-enzyme in many of the chemical reactions in the cell, and has a major role to play in the formation of red blood cells in the bone marrow. The nerve cells and the skin also require it for proper function.

Natural sources: liver, eggs, sea food.

Deficiency manifestations: anaemia, nervous debility, poor concentration, memory loss and lack of energy.

Note: the body's requirements of this vitamin are very small and it should not be taken in excess. It works in conjunction with folic acid. As with all the B vitamins it is better when taken synergistically, that is, in balance with the others in the group.

The main cause of the deficiency diseases seems to be malabsorption in the small intestine, and great attention should be paid to improving the health of the intestines, for example by taking a good supply of yogurt.

If you are using the contraceptive pill, if you smoke, or if you are a vegetarian you may well need extra Vitamin B_{12} in your diet. Strict vegetarians will need to rely on comfrey or kelp, or take this vitamin in supplement form.

Vitamin B Group   Folic Acid

Water soluble.

Measured in micrograms (μg).

Functions: essential for the formation of blood, the growth and division of cells and a healthy digestive process.

Natural sources: green vegetables, liver, milk, yeast, wheatgerm, soya flour.

Deficiency manifestations: diarrhoea, anaemia, depression, glossitis, stomach distension.

Note: folic acid works in conjunction with Vitamin E so it is important to take them together. Together they help the assimilation of pantothenic acid. Coeliacs, users of the contraceptive pill, and pregnant women should pay particular attention to their intake of folic acid.

Vitamin B Group   PABA (Para-aminobenzoic Acid)

Water soluble.

Measured in milligrams (mg).

Form of folic acid.

Very closely related to the B complex, but as it may be synthesised by bacteria in the intestine it is, strictly speaking, not a vitamin.

Functions: helps maintain healthy skin and hair. Essential in the formation of folic acid.

Natural sources: brewer's yeast, whole grains.

Deficiency manifestations: psoriasis, eczema.

Note: this is one of the best sunscreens we can use, so it is an important ingredient in any good ointments for protection against sunburn.

Vitamin B Group   Biotin

Water soluble.

Measured in micrograms (μg).
The intestinal bacteria are able to produce biotin, thus it is not strictly a vitamin.

Functions: essential for the metabolism of proteins, the proper function of the digestive process and in achieving healthy hair.

Natural sources: liver, mushrooms, whole grain rice, brewer's yeast, soya beans, bananas, egg yolks, green vegetables.

Deficiency manifestations: anorexia, depression, debility, muscular pain, anaemia, a possible increase in cholesterol.

Note: raw egg whites seem to be the major enemy of biotin, although food processing and alcohol are close behind.

You will have no deficiency of this substance if you are following the Rowland Remedy Food Guide.

Vitamin B Group Choline

Water soluble.
Measured in milligrams (mg).
The body is able to manufacture its own choline from the amino acid methionine as long as sufficient B_{12} and folic acid are present.

Functions: when combined with inositol it aids the dispersal of fats and fat soluble vitamins throughout the body.

Natural sources: liver, lecithin, brewer's yeast, fish, soya beans, wheatgerm, vegetables.

Deficiency manifestations: loss of memory, poor concentration, senile dementia, poor co-ordination.

Note: extra choline should be added to your diet in the form of lecithin if you consume alcohol or are on the contraceptive pill.

Vitamin B Group Inositol

Water soluble.

Measured in milligrams (mg).

Functions: combined with choline it helps in the dispersal of fats thoughout the body.

Natural sources: liver, lecithin, brewer's yeast, fish, soya beans, whole grains, wheatgerm, vegetables.

Deficiency manifestations: poor concentration, poor memory co-ordination, brain fag, senile dementia.

Note: inositol is sensitive to water, alcohol, caffeine and the contraceptive pill.

Always try to think of inositol with choline, as they have a combined role to play in nature.

Vitamin B_{13} Calcium Orotate

Water soluble.

Measured in milligrams (mg).

Functions: aids cell regeneration, glandular function, proper function of the liver and pancreas. It is linked with metabolising folic acid and Vitamin B_{12}.

Natural sources: milk whey, root vegetables.

Deficiency manifestations: gout, excessive uric acid deposits.

Note: as milk whey is often difficult to obtain, the best source is as a supplement of calcium orotate tablets.

I would recommend Vitamin B_{13} for high blood pressure, as a sports supplement, and for alcoholics who are drying out. It is unquestionably helpful in liver conditions such as hepatitis and cirrhosis.

Vitamin B_{15} Pangamic Acid

Water soluble.

Measured in milligrams (mg).
An anti-oxidant similar in action to Vitamin E.

Functions: helps create healthy blood and tissues, mainly by improving the transportation of oxygen to the cell and improving muscle tissue.

Natural sources: rice bran, maize, oatflakes, wheatgerm.

Deficiency manifestations: brain fag, debility, night cramps, lack of muscle tone.

Note: there is some doubt about whether this substance is essential to life and therefore whether it should have vitamin status, although it is beyond doubt that it is helpful to the body. It certainly helps the blood circulation by improving the supply of oxygen to the cell and, because of this, athletes from all over the world have been taking supplements of pangamic acid for many years now.

It can help with all conditions that require improved circulation, such as diabetes, hypertension, angina, thrombosis, asthma and arthritis. If taken in supplement form, it is important to establish that it is derived from natural sources and not synthetic in origin. If you are on the treatment programme, your intake is guaranteed as this substance is found in foods recommended in the menu, such as bran, oats and wheatgerm.

Vitamin C Ascorbic Acid

Water soluble, thus not stored well by the body.
Measured in milligrams (mg).

Functions: helps to form the intercellular substance collagen necessary for cellular oxidation and reduction. Improves the body's defence mechanisms.

Natural sources: citrus fruits, blackcurrants, strawberries, green vegetables, potatoes, cauliflower.

Deficiency manifestations: scurvy, skin diseases, bleeding gums, sensitive mouth and gums, capillary fragility.

Note: although Vitamin C is probably the best commonly known vitamin there is still much research being done to determine whether high doses might be useful in the prevention and cure of diseases hitherto not associated with the vitamin, such as cancer.

Vitamin D   Calciferols

Fat soluble.
Calciferol measured in micrograms (μg).
Vitamin D measured in international units (i.u.).
1 μg calciferol = 40 i.u.
Vitamin D is really a complex and has at least 10 associates. Two of the most important ones are D_2 or ergocalciferol, and D_3 or cholecalciferol. D_2 is formed when ultra-violet light is passed over the pro-vitamin, or precursor, ergasterol, which is found in the lower forms of plant life, such as yeasts and fungi. D_3 is formed when ultra-violet light is passed over the pro-vitamin cholesterol, which is found in the skin and other tissues. Vitamin D is often referred to as the 'sun vitamin' because of the need for ultra-violet light in its formation.

Functions: essential for the absorption of calcium and phosphorus, and subsequent utilisation for bone growth by regulating the calcium levels in the blood.

Natural sources: fish, dairy products, cod liver oil.

Deficiency manifestations: rickets, soft bones, poor teeth, skeletal deformities.

Note: a very important vitamin for any programme dealing with a degenerative disease. Vitamin D works closely with Vitamin A. I favour cod liver oil and sunlight as the best source of this vitamin.

Vitamin E

Fat soluble.

Measured in international units (i.u.) or milligrams (mg).
d-α tocopherol 1 mg = 1.49 i.u.
d-α tocopheryl acetate 1 mg = 1.36 i.u.
d-α tocopheryl acid succinate 1 mg = 1.21 i.u.
dl-α tocopherol 1 mg = 1.1 i.u.
dl-α tocopheryl acetate 1 mg = 1 i.u.
dl-α tocopheryl acid succinate 1 mg = 0.89 i.u.
The naturally-occurring tocopherols have the prefix d.
The synthetic tocopherols have the prefix dl.
Tocopherol is the alcoholic form.
Tocopheryl is the ester form.

Functions: improves blood circulation, prevents and dissolves blood clots. Acts as an antioxidant in the body, protecting the polyunsaturated fats in the cell walls from peroxidation, thus essential to all life processes.

Natural sources: wheatgerm, green vegetables, vegetable oils, legumes, peanuts, wheatgerm oil.

Deficiency manifestations: poor circulation and fatigue are two signs, but a deficiency will manifest itself in many different diseases associated with degeneration of the body.

Note: Vitamin E has long been known as the anti-sterility vitamin. Care should be taken not to take too much if you are inclined to high blood pressure. If you are on a treatment programme you will be receiving enough.

Vitamin K

Fat soluble.
Synthesised by bacterial activity in the intestine.

Functions: essential to the formation of the factors associated with the clotting of blood.

Natural sources: liver, green vegetables, dairy produce, vegetable oils, soya beans.

Deficiency manifestations: slow clotting of blood and lack of prothrombin.

Note: this vitamin is found in abundance and you can be sure of receiving your body requirements from a mixed diet.

11 Minerals and Trace Elements

Calcium Symbol Ca Atomic Weight 40

There is a greater weight of calcium in the body than of any other mineral and most of it is in the bones and teeth. It is essential for their strong growth and maintenance. It is equally necessary for sound sleep and strong nerves, an undersupply often resulting in muscle spasms and cramp. Adequate Vitamin A must be available for calcium to be assimilated. Calcium has a balanced relationship with magnesium and phosphorus (see below for details of these minerals).

Sources: milk and milk products, cheeses, sardines, nuts, beans, green vegetables. Dolomite tablets (calcium and magnesium in a correct balance) and bonemeal tablets taken with Vitamin A provide good supplements.

Chlorine Symbol Cl Atomic Weight 35.5

As Chlorides

Associated with sodium and potassium, it is required to keep the body fluid's near-neutrality. Chlorine as hydrochloric acid in the stomach aids the digestion of food.

Sources: an excess, in the form of sodium chloride, is more likely than a deficiency (see also sodium below).

As Chlorinated Water Supply

Chlorine is used to destroy bacteria. If the excess chlorine is not removed by boiling, it can reduce Vitamin E levels and useful bacteria in the stomach. This can be remedied by taking supplements of Vitamin E and taking plenty of yogurt.

Chromium Symbol Cr Atomic Weight 52

Chromium is essential to the body's utilisation of carbohydrates. There is evidence to support the theory that diabetes may be caused by a deficiency of this element, perhaps by reducing the tissue response to insulin.

Sources: meat, shellfish, chicken, whole grains, seeds, brewer's yeast. Multi-mineral supplements contain chromium.

Cobalt Symbol Co Atomic Weight 59

Cobalt is contained in Vitamin B_{12} which is the term used to describe a number of cobalamin compounds. These have proved useful in the treatment of pernicious anaemia.

Sources: cobalt as Vitamin B_{12} is found only in food of animal origin and deficiencies, though very rare, may occur in strict vegetarians. Supplements are available and Vitamin B_{12} is normally included in a B complex supplement.

Copper Symbol Cu Atomic Weight 64

Copper is a constituent of all human tissues, with the highest concentrations in the brain, liver, kidneys, heart and pancreas. It is essential for the metabolism of iron in the synthesis of haemoglobin and for the utilisation of Vitamin C and of the amino acid tyrosine. It maintains energy by aiding effective iron absorption.

Most foods contain traces of this element, so deficiency is rare.

Sources: dried beans, peas, prunes, wholewheat, calf and beef liver, sea food.

Fluorine Symbol F Atomic Weight 19

This element belongs to the same group as chlorine, bromine and iodine. It is widely distributed in human tissues, with the highest concentrations found in the teeth and bones. It improves the resistance of the tooth enamel to acids, thus reducing dental caries.

Fluorides are readily absorbed but only slowly excreted in the urine, and so can cause cumulative toxicity. An excess can mottle the teeth.

Sources: sea food. In many areas, there is controlled addition of fluoride to the drinking water (1 p.p.m.). Before taking additional fluoride you should check with your water authority to find out what the level in your area is.

Iodine Symbol I Atomic Weight 127

This element belongs to the same group as chlorine, bromine and fluorine. It is concentrated in the body in the thyroid gland and influences its activity, thus controlling the metabolism. It provides energy and promotes growth, healthy hair, skin and nails.

Iodides are rapidly absorbed and rapidly excreted in the urine but the thyroid is capable of absorbing enough for its requirements very quickly.

Solutions of iodine are used externally as disinfectants.

Sources: iodine is widely distributed in nature, as metallic iodides, in very low concentrations.

Iron   Symbol Fe   Atomic Weight 56

As an element essential to the production of haemoglobin, it is vital to life. Most of the body's iron is found in the blood (as haemoglobin), but it is also needed for muscle pigment (myoglobin) and certain enzymes. The liver, spleen and bone marrow contain iron.

The assimilation of iron requires an adequate presence of the elements copper, cobalt and manganese, and also Vitamin C.

Anaemia is normally associated with iron deficiency.

Sources: liver, kidneys, red meat, egg, oatmeal, nuts, beans. Iron supplements should be the organic acid salts, e.g. gluconate, fumarate or palmitate for best assimilation. Iron salts of inorganic acids, e.g. iron sulphate, are less well assimilated and can be harmful to Vitamin E. The iron must be in the reduced ferrous state; in the oxidised ferric state the iron cannot be absorbed.

Magnesium   Symbol Mg   Atomic Weight 24

Magnesium is essential for the stability of the neuro-muscular system, but in high concentrations it can act as a depressant. It is necessary also for healthy muscle since the muscle enzymes cannot metabolise sugar without it.

It is needed for the assimilation of calcium and phosphorus. A balance between calcium and magnesium exists in a ratio of approximately 2:1 in the body, and an excess of either should be avoided. Magnesium deficiency may cause the deposition of calcium in the soft tissues.

Vitamin B_6 is essential for normal levels of magnesium in the blood and tissues, and magnesium activates many enzymes containing Vitamin B_6. Neither nutrient can function in the absence or deficiency of the other.

Sources: lemons, grapefruit, nuts, apples, green vegetables. If supplements are to be taken, they are best in the form of salts of organic acids rather than magnesium sulphate, because magnesium is absorbed only with difficulty in the gastro-intestinal tract – to the extent, in fact, that it acts as a laxative.

Manganese Symbol Mn Atomic Weight 55

This is an essential trace element, related to vanadium and chromium, found widely in human tissue, particularly in blood, liver, kidney, pancreas and hair. It is necessary for the utilisation of important B vitamins and the function of the central nervous system. It affects the function of the pancreas and a lack of it can lower the glucose tolerance level. It is an essential co-factor in the function of many enzymes. A high calcium and phosphorus intake requires extra manganese.

Sources: nuts, green leaf vegetables, whole grain cereals, oats, rye, peas, beans, dried fruits, raspberries and tea. Manganese is available in synthetic form in mineral supplements.

Molybdenum Symbol Mo Atomic Weight 96

An essential trace element, related to chromium, and present in soils and sea water. It aids in carbohydrate and fat metabolism and there are indications that the presence of molybdenum improves the utilisation of iron.

Sources: vegetables, wheatgerm, fish and other marine-based foods including kelp and sea salt. Synthetic supplements are not recommended because of the possibility of toxicity.

Phosphorus Symbol P Atomic Weight 31

Phosphorus is necessary to the life process in every body cell and for the growth and maintenance of good teeth and bones. The intake must be balanced with the intake of calcium otherwise the excess is excreted as calcium-phosphorus salts, depleting the body's reserve of calcium.

Too much iron and magnesium in food can reduce the assimilation of phosphorus by precipitation of insoluble phosphates in the intestine.

Phosphorus aids in the metabolism of fats and starches and in the assimilation of niacin.

Sources: fish, poultry, meat liver, brewer's yeast, lecithin, eggs, nuts. These should be taken in conjunction with calcium-rich foods.

Potassium Symbol K Atomic Weight 39

The elements potassium and sodium regulate the body's water balance. With the element chlorine, as chloride ion, they maintain the body fluids' near-neutrality. An excess of either potassium or sodium is undesirable, leading to an upset in the body fluid blance.

Potassium activates many enzymes essential for good nerve and muscle function and is necessary also for converting carbohydrates into energy or into body starch (glycogen) for storage.

Sources: vegetables, fruits, whole grains, nuts and meats. Potassium is fairly widely distributed in foods and the requirements should be adequately covered by a well-balanced diet. Remember, though, that a high intake of salt can result in a high potassium loss, as can prolonged periods of mental and physical stress.

Selenium Symbol Se Atomic Weight 79

This element belongs to the same group as sulphur. It is

essential to life and widely distributed in tissues, blood and the main organs.

Selenium is synergistic with Vitamin E in preventing ageing and the hardening of tissues. Liver necrosis and muscular dystrophy may be associated with a selenium deficiency, though this rarely occurs on a good diet.

Sources: tuna, herring, brewer's yeast, wheatgerm, bran, onions, cabbage, tomatoes.

Sodium Symbol Na Atomic Weight 23

See potassium, above, for importance of sodium-potassium balance. Instances of high blood pressure are often associated with an excess of sodium.

Sources: Sodium is so widely distributed in foods, particularly in convenience foods, that the daily intake is more than likely to be in excess of requirements. In abnormal conditions, however, for example when prolonged exposure to heat or long periods of physical exercise result in excessive perspiration, too much sodium may be lost from the body. Additional salt must be taken under these circumstances to prevent heat exhaustion.

Sulphur Symbol S Atomic Weight 32

Sulphur is ingested mainly in the form of sulphur-containing amino acids, e.g. methionine, cysteine and cystine. Methionine is very important as a basis for the synthesis of many essential compounds in the body. The sulphur-containing amino acids are essential for the production of tissue proteins, e.g. keratin, which keeps the nails, skin and hair healthy. They are also involved in the detoxification of aromatic compounds such as benzene.

Sulphur is used as a bactericide in ointments.

Sources: beef, beans, eggs, fish, cabbage.

Vanadium **Symbol V** **Atomic Weight 51**

An essential trace element present in soils and sea water. Its essential role is thought to be the control of formation of cholesterol deposits in the arteries.

Sources: fish and other marine-based foods, including kelp and sea salt. Although excess vanadium is rapidly excreted from the body, synthetic supplements are not recommended because of the possibility of toxicity.

Zinc **Symbol Zn** **Atomic Weight 65**

Whole blood contains a significant quantity of zinc, mainly in the red cells. An adequate supply is necessary for the action of at least twenty enzymes, one of them, in the retina of the eye, being responsible for Vitamin A metabolism (one type of night blindness appears to be due to a zinc deficiency).

High concentrations of zinc are found in the pancreas: it is released at the same time as insulin and appears to prolong its action.

Zinc deficiency can result from a diet high in phosphorus which impairs zinc absorption. Growth and sexual development can be affected, resistance to infection can be lowered, healing impaired and a skin condition similar to psoriasis can result.

Sources: shellfish, lamb, pork, brewer's yeast, pumpkin seeds, eggs. Supplements are available and zinc salts such as gluconate, lactate and citrate are preferred to salts of inorganic acids such as sulphate.

12 Foodstuffs

Bran

Bran is the hard, outer skin of the wheat grain. Although it contains significant quantities of protein, carbohydrate, calcium and iron they have little nutritional value as bran is indigestible in the human alimentary tract. It is, however, this very property which gives it a value as a good source of dietary fibre which, by speeding the passage of waste materials through the bowel, helps to minimise constipation.

Bran is frequently included in weight-reducing diets because of its water retention property which gives a feeling of a full stomach.

Cider Apple Vinegar

Cider apple vinegar, or cider vinegar, contains many different health-giving properties which are not to be found in malt or wine, the other two popular forms of vinegar. It is for this reason that I recommend the use of it whilst you are on your health programme, not only on the table but also for adding as one of the ingredients to your special baths.

Cider apple vinegar is so called because it is made solely from apples, which are naturally high in potassium and minerals such as phosphorus, magnesium, calcium, iron, fluorine and chlorine. Bacteria, which occur naturally, combine with the alcohol to produce a natural acetic acid which has a high mineral content.

The process of manufacture dates back many centuries and was a particularly favourite food in the monasteries where documents show that it was in use both as a food and a medicine well over a thousand years ago. As a food, its high potassium content is beneficial, although the monks, of course, would have been unaware of the reason for its good effect on the body.

As a medicine, often combined with honey as a digestive aid, it counters the blood's increased alkaline reaction to stress and to too many rich foods.

Muesli

In the early twentieth century, the Swiss dietitian, Dr Bircher-Benner, thought that one should start the day with a highly nutritious breakfast that was easy to prepare and had the health-giving properties of fibre, natural nutrients and the properties of milk that are known to help the digestive tract stay healthy. He combined oats, millet and wheat with hazel nuts, almonds and fresh apple and added a little lemon juice with honey and milk to taste. This provided all the nutrients that the body would need to start the day.

Today there are many brands of muesli available in the shops, all of them based on the original concept of Dr Bircher-Benner. You will see from the programme that muesli is used as the base for the Rowland Remedy breakfast. However, I do appreciate that some people react badly to muesli and, in these circumstances, I recommend porridge as a base. See below for details of oats.

Oatmeal

Oats are the edible grain from the cereal grass, *Avena sativa*, which is used by herbalists for its muscle- and body-building properties and as a nerve tonic. Oatmeal is one of the most nutritious of the cereals, but surprisingly is not widely used. It has a well balanced protein, fat and carbohydrate content, giving it a high energy value. It is also a useful source of Vitamin B_1 and iron.

Its energy value is best obtained as oatcakes. As porridge, it is easily digested but its energy value per serving is significantly reduced by the dilution with water.

Salads

All the usual vegetable ingredients of a salad, for example lettuce, celery, onions, peppers, tomatoes and cucumber, have a low energy value. The main nutritional value of salads lies in their vitamin A, potassium and iron content and they should always be made up with fresh ingredients.

Sprouting Seeds

Seeds contain the concentrated energy to enable a plant to survive during its early growth. The sprouting seeds contain vitamins and nutrients in a live, growing state, as opposed to vegetables and fruits that have been harvested for an unknown period, are no longer fresh and have deteriorated to some degree.

Sprouting seeds can be cultivated at home and suitable seeds and instructions can be purchased at health food stores.

One of my favourite sprouting seeds is mung bean sprouts. These are exceptionally high in nutrients, particularly potassium. The nutrients are in an easily absorbable form during the period that the beans are sprouting and they are thus a highly desirable food.

Vegetables, Root and Tuber

The reason I recommend the use of root vegetables in salads is for their energy and nutritive values, the roots being the plants' storehouse of sugars and starches. There are also many health properties ascribed to roots. Beetroot, for instance, is reputed to be an excellent food for the red blood corpuscles and is the reason why it is the basis for a naturopathic approach to treating various forms of cancer, with the juice from 1.5 kg of the fresh roots being consumed daily by patients who are on special diets for this condition.

Carrots are another favourite root of mine, the juice being of great value in many conditions, due to the concentrations of the precursor β-carotene and other nutrients. They can be of help to people who have arthritis and also to those who suffer from conditions such as obesity, high blood pressure, colitis and poor eyesight, among others. The maximum benefits can be obtained from the carrot by extracting the juice or shredding the raw flesh as part of a salad.

Another well known root is horseradish (*Armoracia rusticana*), a highly concentrated food which stimulates the appetite by aiding the secretion of gastric juices. It has the reputation of being a solvent for any excess of mucus in the system, so it is especially useful to include in your diet when you have a cold or catarrh, and perhaps asthma. Do not eat too much, however, as it can be irritating to the kidneys and bladder.

The Jerusalem artichoke is the tuber of the *Helianthus tuberosus* plant and is a very worthwhile food, particularly for diabetics who have to watch the overall amount of carbohydrate in their food.

Onions are of special interest to us on this health programme as they are not only high in potassium but also have undisputed antiseptic properties and are helpful in draining the cavities of mucus, so helping in the detoxification sections of our treatment.

Parsnips (*Pastinaca sativa*) should be included in your diet, cooked only briefly.

Sweet potatoes are the edible tubers of *Batatas batatas*. They are a rich source of vitamins and minerals, being particularly rich in phosphorus and potassium. They are easily digested and have beneficial effects on people with delicate digestive processes, stomach ulcers and inflamed conditions such as colitis. They can be prepared for eating in much the same way as the white potato.

The white potato is the edible tuber of *Solanum tuberosum* and is so well known that it need not be dealt with in any detail, except to say that I have often recommended the juice of the white potato to be drunk three times daily on an empty stomach for stomach ulcers. This was a recommendation of a friend of mine, Dr A. Vogel, made some years ago when he was paying me a visit and I have passed on the advice to the great benefit of a lot of people.

Water

In view of the fact that our body weight is made up of 70% fluid, I feel that we should pay some attention to the type of water that we drink.

Water, being nature's solvent, is essential to the proper working of the body. It is necessary to have an adequate (regular) intake of water for the kidneys to work efficiently, i.e. 1-1.5 litres as liquid and approximately 1 litre as food. The digestive process relies on water to work efficiently and so does the skin for its many functions. Due to the regular loss of fluid by the body (about 2 litres per day) it is important to replace this amount on a daily basis.

In most western countries, the tap water is safe due to the bactericides that are added, but I nevertheless recommend a home water-filter system which may be purchased at very low cost. It will give you good clear water for drinking or for making herbal teas, or for ice cubes or for cooking. It removes the chalk, scum, taint and the dissolved gases that we do not want and leaves behind the minerals and trace elements that are so important to good health.

The alternative is bottled mineral waters that are now becoming popular all over the world: you will be drinking water with healthy properties, at the same time eliminating the need to drink from the local supply.

The EEC rules for classifying a mineral water require that nothing can be added or taken away; the only exceptions are the separation of the unstable elements, such as iron and sulphur compounds. This may be achieved by filtering or decanting methods with the strict proviso that the basic composition of the water is not altered. They also require that the water be from an underground source that is bacteriologically pure and of constant composition.

All water contains nitrate, which in excess can be harmful to babies as it can change to nitrite in the body and interfere with the transfer of oxygen in the bloodstream. To obviate this, the EEC permits a maximum level of nitrate of 50 mg per litre for all waters whether tap or bottled.

The sodium content is also controlled at a maximum of 175 mg per litre, as it is generally accepted that high salt levels are undesirable.

You will have gathered that I am keen on having a home filter system and using bottled mineral waters whenever possible. Here are details of some mineral waters available on the market.

Apollinaris (Bad Neuenahr, West Germany) Named after St Apollinaris, it has a naturally sparkling, slightly alkaline, taste with a high mineral content.

Ashbourne (Derbyshire, Peak District, England) Due to the fact that the UK has no naturally sparkling springs, this water is available both in its still form and also artificially carbonated.
Badoit (St Galmier, France) A lightly sparkling water from deep in the Alps with a high calcium and magnesium content. Refer to pp.108 and 111 for more information on these minerals.
Contrex (France) This is a still water, high in minerals, which also has natural diuretic properties.
Evian (Mont Blanc, France) A still water with a low mineral content.
Highland Spring (Perthshire, Scotland) Like Ashbourne water, this is available in its natural still form or artificially carbonated.
Malvern (Malvern Hills, England) Available in both still and carbonated forms.
Perrier (Vergeze, South of France) A favourite all over the world. It has a natural sparkle created by past volcanic activity which has dissolved the gases in Perrier which includes traces of xenon, crypton, argon, neon and helium.
San Pellegrina (Italy) This has a high mineral content and has been artificially carbonated to make an ideal dining accompaniment.
Spa (Belgium) A popular low-mineral water that is available in its naturally sparkling form or in a still form for regular use.
Vichy Celestins (France) Has a high sodium bicarbonate content which has made it a popular guest at a rich meal. I have many patients who order this water by the crate because they are so impressed by the aid it has given their digestive system.
Vichy St Yorre (France) Has a slight sparkle and is gaining popularity as a top quality table water.
Vittel (France) A still water which has an overall low mineral content but is high in calcium and magnesium and

therefore has all the benefits of these minerals (see pp.108 and 111).
Volvic (Auvergne Mountains, France) A still water, low in minerals.

Wheatgerm

Wheatgerm is the part of the grain that is needed for the wheat to germinate. It is the life force of the grain and a rich source of concentrated nutrients. It contains Vitamins A, E and the B group, also copper, magnesium, manganese, calcium and phosphorus as well as other trace elements. It is thus included in the breakfast programme.

It is usually available in two forms. The first is the completely unprocessed raw form, which is certainly the best source of the nutrients but which is more susceptible to rancidity. This form should be refrigerated for storage and used up quickly.

Probably the safer form is stabilised, or toasted, wheatgerm which keeps for a much longer period and has a pleasanter taste. It also should be refrigerated once opened, preferably in an airtight container.

Wholemeal, Wholewheat, Wheatmeal Flour

There is often a degree of confusion about the different types of brown flour available. In the main there are two types of brown flour: a) wholewheat, wholemeal or 100% wholemeal and b) wheatmeal.

You can immediately see where the confusion arises, especially when the prefix 'stoneground' appears on many packets of flour on the shelves today. So let us take a closer look. Wholewheat, wholemeal and 100% wholemeal are all whole grain flour using 100% of the wheat grain, including the bran and the wheatgerm. The word to be looking for is 'whole'.

Wheatmeal, on the other hand, has either 15% or 19% of the bran (depending on which type of wheat is used) removed to give a smoother flour. It is therefore better for you than white flour but not so nutritious as wholewheat flour.

Many of the flours on sale are described as being stone-ground. This means that the flour was made by rotating two stones at slow speeds. This process has many advantages over the newer steel roller mills in that the stones maintain the grain at a lower temperature and therefore preserve the heat-sensitive nutrients, such as Vitamin E, for the consumer's benefit.

Addresses

Letters to the author will be most welcome and should be addressed to: The Naturopathic Private Clinic, 76 Victoria Road East, Thornton Cleveleys, Lancashire FY5 5HH (0253 853482). Residents in Eire are advised to contact the author: c/o Herbal Health, 5 Ardee Road, Rathmines, Dublin 6.

General Council and Register of Consultant Herbalists, Villa Merlyn, 18 Elgin Road, Talbot Road, Bournemouth BH4 9NL.

Herb Society of America, 300 Massachusetts Avenue, Boston, Massachusetts 02115, USA.

National Institute of Medical Herbalists, School of Herbal Medicine, 148 Forest Road, Tunbridge Wells, Kent.

Queensland Herb Society, 23 Greenmount Avenue, Holland Park, Brisbane, Queensland, Australia.

Tasmanian Herb Society, 12 Delta Avenue, Taroona, Tasmania 7006, Australia.

INDEX

Numbers in *italics* refer to illustrations